CONVERSING WITH UNCERTAINTY

Relational Perspectives Book Series

Stephen A. Mitchell, Series Editor

Volume 1
Rita Wiley McCleary
*Conversing with Uncertainty:
Practicing Psychotherapy in a Hospital Setting*

In Preparation
Lewis Aron
Interpretation and Subjectivity

Emmanuel Ghent
Process and Paradox

Charles Spezzano
Affects and Therapeutic Action

Donnel Stern
Unformulated Experience

Rita Wiley McCleary

CONVERSING WITH UNCERTAINTY

Practicing Psychotherapy in a Hospital Setting

with a
Foreword by Stephen A. Mitchell

and an
Afterword by Glen O. Gabbard

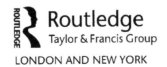

Routledge
Taylor & Francis Group

LONDON AND NEW YORK

First published 1992 by The Analytic Press, Inc.

This edition published 2015 by Routledge
2 Park Square, Milton Park, Abingdon, Oxon OX14 4RN
711 Third Avenue, New York, NY 10017, USA

Routledge is an imprint of the Taylor &Francis Group, an informa business

Set in Korinna by Lind Graphics, Inc., Upper Saddle River, NJ

Library of Congress Cataloging-in-Publication Data

McCleary, Rita Wiley.
 Conversing with uncertainty : practicing psychotherapy in a
 hospital setting / Rita Wiley McCleary, with a foreword by Stephen
 A. Mitchell and an afterword by Glen O. Gabbard.
  p. cm.—Relational Perspectives Book Series ; v. 1
 Includes bibliographical references and index.
 ISBN 0-88163-148-5
 1. Psychotherapy—Case studies. 2. Psychiatric hospital care—
Case studies. 3. Psychotherapist and patient—Case studies.
4. Psychotherapy—Philosophy. 5. McCleary, Rita Wiley.
6. Psychotherapy. I. Title.
 [DNLM: 1. Inpatients—psychology.   WM 420 M478c]
RC465.M39 1992
616.89'14—dc20
DNLM/DLC
for Library of Congress   92-17730
                                                                            CIP

ISBN-13: 978-0-88163-148-7 (hbk)

To my parents, Dick and Francesca

ACKNOWLEDGMENTS

In *Educating the Reflective Practitioner*, Donald Schön (1987) argued that "the paradox of learning a really new competence is this: that a student cannot at first understand what he needs to learn, can learn it only by educating himself, and can educate himself only by beginning to do what he does not yet understand" (p. 93). While in many respects Schön's depiction of learning-in-action inspired the following case study, I think that here he overstates his point. To agree that I could learn to be a good psychotherapist only through my own practicing is not to detract in the slightest from the indispensable support, guidance, and constructive criticism from others that I gratefully received, depended on, and used.

My first thanks goes to Kay, the adolescent inpatient who tolerated my often clumsy efforts to be her psychotherapist and whose talking back yielded insights into how I was treating her that I could never have gained from a textbook. For all her very real difficulties in living, I remember her intelligence, humor, and admirable—if, at times, exasperating—stubborness. Kay and I were both lucky to find ourselves on an adolescent unit at State Psychiatric Hospital. By their example, clinical staff members taught me the value of team work in a hospital setting and positively contributed to Kay's treatment.

At the Chicago School of Professional Psychology, where this book germinated as a dissertation, Dennis McCaughan, my advisor, lent me his remarkable capacity to make sense of problematic materials and shape them into a reflective case study. He balanced his strong commitment to psychoanalytic inquiry with an equally deep appreciation for new and often unexpected ways of under-standing. His love of ideas never lost touch with the complex situations that my own ideas attempted to approximate. Very rarely in my many years as a student did I have the good fortune to study with someone at once so talented and generous.

Other colleagues and de facto advisors whose comments and encouragement have helped me include Margaret Browning, Kirsten Dahl, Lynn Reiser, Donna Robinson, David Smigelskis, Herb Wein-stein, and Lee Weiss. I owe special thanks to Richard Davis for his uncomplaining willingness to read and respond to innumerable drafts, and whose unflagging confidence in the project sustained me during those long hours of figuring out what I was trying to say.

I felt honored when The Analytic Press accepted my book for publication and was subsequently awed by the editors' generosity. Paul Stepansky, Editor-in-Chief, always made himself available as both a sounding board and source of complementary ideas that sparked my own. Similarly, John Kerr, who read both the initial and final drafts, provided stimulating and astute comments. Without Eleanor Starke Kobrin, TAP's Managing Editor, the book would never have seen the light of day. She coached me in the finer points of Wordstar and gently assured me that I, like other new authors, could surely compile an index.

Last but not least, I want to extend special thanks to Merton Gill. Often as I struggled through the writing of this case, I thought of it as a psychoanalysis of my ideas. The confidence and stamina required to persist in such often disheartening self-scrutiny would not have been possible without his patience, wisdom, and example.

CONTENTS

FOREWORD

Stephen A. Mitchell

With certain kinds of experiences, the first time is always memorable, whether it is good or bad, a triumph or a disaster. These are kinds of experiences for which one is completely unprepared, experiences unlike anything else that has come before. Doing psychotherapy is one of those experiences. There is nothing else quite like it, and there is no way to appreciate that until you are in the middle of it for the first time.

My first experiences doing psychotherapy took place at a large, prominent teaching hospital in New York City at the beginning of my psychology internship. As in most training institutions, we arrived on July 1 and were assigned our patients, in my case, two community service inpatients and several outpatients. Although there were supervisors and administrative staff to help us, we suddenly had primary responsibility for the lives of those assigned to our care. With an allowance of some time to get to know them (a few days!), we were expected to make decisions having major implications for their lives: privileges and restrictions within the hospital, privileges to leave the hospital, discharge, disposition, and so on.

I was reasonably prepared, in comparison with my peers. I had had two solid years of course work in clinical psychology. I had studied, fairly extensively, theories of personality, abnormal psychology, and theories of psychotherapy. I had studied, adminis-

Stephen A. Mitchell, Ph.D. is Faculty and Supervisor, New York University Postdoctoral Program in Psychotherapy and Psychoanalysis, and Editor of *Psychoanalytic Dialogues: A Journal of Relational Perspectives.*

tered, and learned to evaluate projective tests like the Rorschach, which provide a unique and highly provocative window into the workings of the mind and the textures of subjective experience. I had also had some practical experience working as a nurse's aide on a psychiatric unit of another hospital. I had gone through the typical shocks when immersed in psychotic experience and behavior for the first time: the spookiness, the subtle pervasiveness of the terror, the startling realization that the only reliable way to distinguish the staff from the patients was often that the former possessed keys that unlocked the doors to the ward.

But having primary therapeutic responsibility for my own patients was something else entirely. Many of these people suffered extraordinary pain. They were often either desperate or, alternately, calmly pursuing courses of thought or action that were bound to be calamitous for them. The sense of responsibility was quite overwhelming. It seemed as if it would require years of study, reflection, and consultation for me to be able reasonably to make decisions that I was now called on to make everyday.

One of my most vivid memories of that time in my life was the dread with which I approached "morning rounds," particularly on Monday mornings. I would now hear what my patients had done over the weekend, and there was the clear sense that I was somehow responsible for their actions and would be called on to account for them and do something about them. Some of the people under my care were abusive, verbally and physically; some were involved in sneaking and selling drugs (including other patients in their clientele); and some were deeply, suicidally depressed. I generally had found it enough of a challenge to account for my own experience and behavior; understanding, accounting for, and making decisions in relation to their's seemed impossible.

I felt even worse for the first-year psychiatric residents who were beginning their training at the same time. They had 10 or 12 inpatients to my two and many other responsibilities. They also had much less training and had been exposed much less to ideas and theories that might have been useful in sorting out their impressions. They had a tool, however, that made managing the behavior of those in their care much easier—medication. At the same time as I developed serious doubt about the value of much of the sedating and mood-altering medication for the patients, I could vividly appreciate how deeply soothing for the therapists was the control that medication gave them over those whose desperate, chaotic lives were now in their hands.

Reading *Conversing With Uncertainty* by Rita McCleary evoked these memories in a particularly exciting way. This is a story of her struggles in her initial encounters with patients, particularly with one extremely troubled, compelling, adolescent girl. What makes this account especially fascinating and far reaching in its implications is that the tool McCleary wrestles with to help both her patient and herself is not medication, or administrative formulas, but clinical theory. It is ideas, understanding that she turns to for help. And the ideas that are available, in existing clinical theories, *do* help her; they also let her down.

In *Conversing With Uncertainty*, the reader is allowed an unusual access to very personal and private conversations between the author and the theorists she turns to for help. She uses, in turn, Masterson's guide for understanding and treating borderlines, the concept of "projective identification" as it has become popularized in recent clinical theorizing, and systems-theory approaches to the hospital milieu. She uses these concepts very much in the sense that Winnicott describes the "use" of an object: she picks them up, bends them to her own experiences, bends her own experiences to fit them, takes them apart, rearranges them, discards them, goes back to them over and over. She makes them hers. Although she is rigorous and extremely conscientious, the major value in this story is not its scholarship or comprehensiveness in the treatment of these ideas, but the deeply personal way they are approached. McCleary is startlingly honest in her account of the personal resonances and meanings of these concepts for her, in her hopes and disillusionments in them, in her uses and abuses of theory.

Perhaps the greatest irony, absurdity, and cruelty of the mental health care system in the United States is that the most difficult patients are treated by the most inexperienced therapists. People with the most complex psychological problems, compounded by social and economic hardship and chronically traumatic backgrounds and living conditions, are the patients first encountered by beginning therapists. This contributes to making McCleary's struggle to find a way to help her patient particularly poignant and wrenching. But the issues with which McCleary grapples are felt not only by beginning clinicians and are not limited only to work with more disturbed patients. Psychoanalysis, an expensive treatment generally available for the socioeconomically privileged and high functioning, is, ultimately, also complex, mysterious, and harrowing. Our responsibility for the patient, and our need to know, both for them and for us, is often painfully great. Our theories are woefully inadequate to the task.

We are living in a time when there is a general crisis of authority in virtually every domain of public and private life. Standard ideologies and traditional formulas have become increasingly irrelevant, and new solutions appear, attain popularity, and vanish with increasing rapidity. This is certainly true in the realm of psychoanalytic ideas. Even 20 years ago there was a clearly identifiable mainstream for those interested in lots of company in a safe, well-worn channel that avoided shoals and rapids. Today there are many compelling, competing schools of psychoanalytic thought; even those who claim to be in the mainstream are so different, one from the other, that there is no longer any course that can claim a meaningful, substantive consensus on important clinical issues encountered in our daily work with patients. There is less a mainstream than a swamp. The sense of objectivity, singular truth, and scriptural reverence for theory that characterized previous generations of psychoanalysts and psychotherapists is no longer really possible for those of us working today.

One popular response to the general disillusionment with theory has been an explicit or implicit antitheoretical attitude sometimes approaching a more general anti-intellectualism. Not only does theory fail to save us, we are told, it gets in our way. Steadfastness in the face of ignorance is the mark of the good clinician; theory is for the fainthearted. One of the more dramatic expressions of this sentiment was Bion's anguished injunction to destroy his books immediately after reading them. It is terrifying but essential to face uncertainty head-on; theory is a seductive buffer and salve to our anxiety. We are better off without it. The analyst should engage the patient with "neither memory or desire" (Bion, 1967) and, presumably, without theory.

McCleary, by contrast, takes theory very seriously, but not too seriously. She asks a lot from the authors she engages but gives them a lot also. She takes what she can from a set of theoretical concepts and then moves on. She is respectful without being deferential. She is not interested just in the truth value of a concept (how well it helps you understand something "out there"), but also in the utility value of a concept (its impact on you and the way you function "out there" thinking in that particular way).

An additional feature of this volume is the afterword by Glen Gabbard, M.D., Director of the C. F. Menninger Memorial Hospital. In Gabbard's commentary on McCleary's account of and reflection upon her own experience, we get another perspective on the complex relationship between theory and clinical process. Whereas McCleary is immersed in difficult clinical problems for the first time, Gabbard has had many years of experience working with similar patients in similar situations and has been a central and original contributor in developing a framework for understanding and working analytically with such patients. Gabbard has found theoretical concepts that work for him (he places considerable emphasis on "projective identification" as applied to group phenomena); he brings an illuminating perspective to McCleary's experiences by organizing them through his own framework. The reader, however, will appreciate McCleary's searching challenge to the finality of any theory and, it is hoped, apply it to Gabbard's current synthesis as well.

It is a commonplace for writers to report a depressive experience upon completion of a book. I have the sense that that state may have a particular quality for writers of clinical theory. It is hard enough to have to declare a book finished. While you are working on it, it is open, alive, still pregnant with unrealized possibilities. Once it is sent by the publisher to the printer, it is finished, dead, unalterable.

The particular wrinkle for the author of clinical theory is that while the book has stopped, your thinking has gone on. You see your patients the next day, and the inadequacy of the theory to capture new features of the clinical experience is inescapable. You notice something new or something old in a new way. You realize that in writing about one thing, you have neglected other important things. There are two extreme options for dealing with this crisis: standing by the theory and insisting that it does, in fact, explain everything (a common practice) or abandoning theory and starting afresh each time (Bion's radical solution). McCleary helps us fashion a third alternative, crucial for our current needs as clinicians and as theoreticians, in which we can value and use our theories without having to sanctify them. Her approach resonates with Einstein's attitude toward theory in physics: "One thing I have learned in a long life:

that all our science, measured against reality, is primitive and childlike—and yet it is the most precious thing we have" (quoted in Ferris, 1988, p. 15).

Conversing With Uncertainty is the first in a new series of books under the general title "Relational Perspectives in Psychoanalysis." It is a wonderful inaugural volume, both because of its high quality and intrinsic interest and also because it expresses the combination of attitudes toward theory and the relationship between theory and clinical practice that I find most reasonable, useful, and inspiring.

REFERENCES

Bion, W. (1967), Notes on memory and desire. In: *Melanie Klein Today: Developments in Theory and Practice,* Vol. 2, ed. E. Bott Spillius. London: Routledge.
Ferris, T. (1988), *Coming of Age in the Milky Way.* New York: William Morrow.

1

FIRST WORDS

*Life can only be understood backwards, but it must be
lived forwards.*
Søren Kierkegaard, *Either/Or*

When I first saw Kay, she looked larger than life, and she scared me.
She was dressed all in black and outraged. Her hair was black and
spiked up on her head, she had rimmed her blue eyes with black, her
tight jeans and tee shirt were black, and her mood was black. I felt
pale, if not invisible, by comparison and scurried past her room
without stopping to introduce myself. Kay was shouting at the
milieu worker with her that she had no need for hospitalization, that
the "state system" had victimized her, and that she was goddamned
if she could not smoke. I would have sworn at the time that she was
wearing chains (she was not). Back in the nurses' station, I tried to
minimize my nervousness as I listened to staff members grumble
that this kid had an awful lot of baggage to sort through and that her
nose-ring was disgusting. I did not know what to think or say.

   This case study is as much about myself as it is about the
adolescent girl whom I treated for nine of the ten months she
remained hospitalized at the State Psychiatric Hospital. To tell the
story of Kay's intensive, and often intense, psychotherapy is to
reconstruct a relationship that was at least as significant for my

personal and professional development as it was for any improvements in her behavior and capacity to live civilly with others. Our
relationship occasioned, for me, a continuing series of reflections,
formulations, and interventions, each of which informed and transformed my appreciation of what the relationship was about and what
role I played within it. What I hope to convey, by way of my own
example, is how thoroughly and inevitably therapists ground their
ideas in the nitty-gritty exigencies of working with patients.

When I began my psychotherapy practicum at State in July 1985,
I was relatively inexperienced as a therapist, but not without intellectual commitments and fairly strong convictions about how I
should do therapy. More than a decade before, as an undergraduate,
I had read Harry Stack Sullivan's (1953) *The Interpersonal Theory of
Psychiatry* under the tutelage of Eugene Gendlin, and since that
time had pursued a passionate interest in how notions of "self" and
"other" mutually defined themselves. Before deciding to seek clinical training, I had also studied philosophy, writing my thesis on
Merleau-Ponty's (1945) conceptualization of intersubjectivity. I subsequently explored related topics in the areas of biography and
fiction. Once invested in my psychotherapeutic training, I gravitated
toward interpersonal formulations of psychoanalytic treatment, as
represented by Edgar Levenson (1972, 1981, 1982), Merton Gill
(1983, 1985), Irwin Hoffman (1983), and Greenberg and Mitchell
(1983), in addition to Sullivan (1940, 1953, 1954). In short, my
personal predilection and studies came together in a dream of a
future as a psychoanalytic psychotherapist with an interpersonalist
bent.

In important respects, this case study owes a debt to the psychoanalytic theorists I had embraced and can be read as an appreciation
of their relevance to clinical practice. Curiously, however, during
that first panicky moment when I glimpsed Kay, and for many weeks
thereafter, their collective wisdom escaped me. Instead of sagely
appreciating the subtleties of the interpersonal encounter, I tried out
this or that idea or intervention, almost blindly at first. Only very
gradually did I gain a more reflective sense of what seemed to work
and why, and at no time, with the exception of occasional conscious
efforts to "analyze the transference," did I apply directly the concepts of interpersonal psychoanalysis. Still, as I have examined and
reexamined my experiences at State, I have come to regard this
narrative as exemplary of an interactive "structure of inquiry," akin

to what Sullivan, borrowing from anthropology, called "participant observation."

Edgar Levenson (1972) captured a therapist's experience of participant observation—and its difference from more exclusively academic efforts—when he wrote the following:

> It is not the therapist's uncoding of the dynamics that makes the therapy, not his "interpretations" of meaning and purpose, but, rather, his extended participation with the patient. It is not his ability to resist distortion by the patient (transference) or to resist his own temptation to interact irrationally with the patient (countertransference) but, rather, his ability to be trapped, immersed, and participating in a system and then to work his way out [p. 174].

At one level this case study illustrates the particularities of getting caught up in an interpersonal system and what it means to work one's way out. At another level, as I will argue more fully later, I think that writing—and reading—such a case study represents a unique form of reflection on clinical practicing that has especial relevance for psychotherapeutic training.

Because she proved to be so controversial, demanding, and dramatic, I was particularly immersed in my work with Kay. Her baggage, of course, was figurative as well as literal, and several pieces had preceded her arrival. We learned that she was 16 1/2 years old and had been a ward of the state for several years. Her parents (who had divorced by the time she was six and who shuttled her back and forth between them) had physically and emotionally abused her as a child. She had run away from her father repeatedly until he finally gave up his custody of her.

In leaving her father's house for a Children's Aid Society (CAS) group home, it seemed that Kay had jumped from the frying pan into the fire: a child prostitution ring operating out of her placement conscripted her into service at age 14. This fact, which shifted in significance and prominence throughout her hospitalization, lent Kay an exceptional, if not favored, status from the start. Following a successful suit against CAS for mistreatment, the court legally mandated CAS to assume full responsibility for Kay until her 21st birthday, a situation many CAS workers resented. Kay's anger and frequently proclaimed sense of entitlement chafed them, yet they could not dismiss her. As I will recount in greater detail in chapter 2,

Kay had spent a year in a prestigious private institution prior to arriving at State, but her length of stay there was always in question. I had the impression that more than one worker took grim satisfaction in her "demotion" to a state hospital, as if now Kay had gotten what she deserved. [1]

The most shocking piece of information about Kay, received the day before she arrived, on September 29, was recorded by the chief social worker as an entry, called a "passalong" or "PAL," in the unit's informal log. Everyone who worked on the unit, from psychiatric aide to unit chief, relied on this clipboard of handwritten notes to learn up-to-the-minute information about patients, to communicate with one another about unit procedures, and sometimes just to complain. Thus, within hours, everyone on A-2 had read: "Kay Z (new patient) has a lawyer, Katherine Q, who might call and arrange a time to see her. She should be allowed to come—she's defending Kay on charges of sexually abusing minors." An abusive delinquent elicits far less sympathy than a child whom others have abused. Confronted with the ill-defined task of treating this girl, with no empathic identification with her predicament, I felt rudderless and alone.

I think that the nursing and milieu staff also felt overwhelmed by Kay's arrival, but for different reasons. For them she threatened to be the proverbial straw that broke the camel's back. An obnoxious and morally repulsive sex offender brought in through political channels, from far outside the unit's catchment area and at a time when the unit chief had promised—impossibly—to keep the census low, was the last thing the staff wanted. They bitterly complained about being a "dumping ground" for "unmanageable" cases. That Kay was not blond and pretty, as a CAS worker had told us, only made matters worse.

With the distance of time and subsequent developments, I have come to reevaluate the staff's anger at my patient, along with everything else. I have come to recognize that beneath the resentment and disgust (curiously focused on the nose-ring) was enough of a sense of challenge and of pride in the unit's work to keep them minimally engaged. That Kay had previously received treatment on

---

[1] As it happens, I think that not only did Kay receive good care at State but in an important sense she herself felt more at home there. She initially flaunted having rubbed elbows with the wealthy but eventually revealed a profound and painful sense of not belonging.

a well-known private adolescent unit spurred the State staff to prove they could do better. When Kay first arrived, however, what I was aware of and reactive to was the staff's antipathy to a case that (for better or worse) I had claimed as my own. It was only a matter of days before I became angry as well.

Needless to say, Kay was not the only one with baggage. I, too, had a history, albeit far less sordid, as did the unit staff, both collectively and individually, and the various agencies and institutions involved in Kay's care. At the time of Kay's admission I had been at State, on A-2, one of the hospital's three adolescent units, for three months (out of an eventual twelve). I had inherited two patients from the previous year's trainees, one now discharged and the other (my favorite) about to be. If I remember correctly, I anticipated Kay, sight as yet unseen, as my first real patient. Thus, for a variety of reasons, I felt remarkably possessive.

I shared my training on the unit with three third-year psychology graduate students like myself, a fourth-year full-time psychology intern, a string of medical residents, and an occasional trainee in psychodiagnostics, occupational therapy, and the like. After three months I knew my way around and my initial apprehensions about working with "crazy kids" had more or less abated. My early enthusiasm had also waned, however: I had had a run-in with the nurse supervisor that left me in tears, my relationship with my own supervisor seemed off to a rocky start, and the staff, while generally friendly, let me know that trainees were often irritants who hindered as much as helped the patients' hospital course. Any exalted notions I had had of being a primary psychotherapist had faded, and I had fallen back to a more questioning and uncertain position.

In many ways Dennis McCaughan (1985) captured my distress and disorientation as a student of adolescent psychotherapy in his article "Teaching and Learning Adolescent Psychotherapy: Adolescent, Therapist, and Milieu." He noted students' typical lack of preparation for inpatient work; their uneasy, and sometimes hostile, alliance with the milieu staff; their increasing insecurity about their role on the unit; and, most important, their disheartening admission (weeks into the therapy) that "their" patient wants no part of their help:

> The character-disordered adolescent's need to act out as a defense against the recognition of a painful and often tormented inner world

runs counter to the therapist's reflective orientation derived from psychoanalytic models of psychotherapy. Many of these adolescents simply do not want treatment. They resist its frustrations, having organized their lives around the immediate gratification of drugs, promiscuity, and a range of anti-social acts. . . . Novice psychotherapists must contend not only with the emotional responses generated by the adolescent's hostility and impulsiveness, but also with the devaluation of a psychotherapeutic orientation that they have come to prize both professionally and personally [p. 416].

When I first read McCaughan's article, shortly before I began at State, it made me vaguely uneasy, but its accuracy and utility eluded me (not unlike the elusiveness of interpersonal theories of psycho-analysis that I mentioned earlier). When I read McCaughan again, six months later, it occasioned a shock of relieved recognition and, when supplemented by a directed readings course, introduced me to the wide-ranging perspective of milieu therapy. Although this case study is not primarily an *apologia* for milieu therapy, McCaughan's viewpoint convinced me that the story I want to tell here has to include in its broad cast of characters the unit staff, the institutional politics, and my teachers and supervisors, as well as, of course, myself and Kay. In so doing, I am heeding McCaughan's concluding advice that "it is necessary to develop a conceptualization that allows for the integration of the therapist, the adolescent, and the milieu. Without such a conceptualization, attempts at treating the adolescent and teaching the therapist are compromised" (p. 422).

The most exciting development in the midst of my enthusiastic reading of the milieu literature was a newfound awareness that formerly abstract, if attractive, ideas might finally pay off. Not only could I now conceive of a productive working relationship with the staff, for instance, but I could also begin to talk to them about it in a way that vastly improved our rapport. The work of Donald Schön, a professor of urban studies and education at the Massachusetts Institute of Technology, complemented and enhanced this realiza-tion. In *The Reflective Practitioner* (1983) and its sequel, *Educating the Reflective Practitioner* (1987), Schön wove together his own detailed examples of professional practicing, from fields as diverse as engi-neering, town planning, and psychotherapy, as a way of exempli-fying and engaging his reader in what he called "reflection-in-action." Schön's characterization of the "push-me pull-me" of doing and thinking-about-doing has helped me enormously to articulate a sense to my work with Kay that neither discounts the contributions of various ideas I entertained nor glosses over the innumerable times I felt stupid and stuck. Given the extent of his influence on my story's "plot," I will present Schön's thesis in some detail before turning to more specific introductions of the chapters that follow.

Schön (1983) began by inviting all professionals to really look at what they do, to recognize that, contrary to popular opinion, their primary activity is problem-*setting*, not problem-*solving*:

> In real-world practice, problems do not present themselves to the practitioner as givens. They must be constructed from the materials of problematic situations which are puzzling, troubling, and uncertain. In order to convert a problematic situation to a problem, a practitioner must do a certain kind of work. He must make sense of an uncertain situation that initially makes no sense [p. 40].

A novice practitioner, of course, will be at a loss as to where to start. Quoting a master architect, a problem-designer par excellence, Schön (1983) advised, "You should begin with a discipline, even if it's arbitrary . . . you can always break it open later" (p. 85). Using a discipline and making a move, the experienced practitioner, as well as the student, must then listen for "back talk," the frequently surprising way in which a problematic situation responds to and influences our ongoing activity. Problem designing is a "conversation with materials" (p. 78) that Schön characterized more fully as follows:

> At the same time that the inquirer tries to shape the situation to his frame, he must hold himself open to the situation's back-talk. He must be willing to enter into new confusions and uncertainties. Hence, he must adopt a kind of double-vision. He must act in accordance with the view he has adopted, but he must recognize that he can always break it open later, indeed *must* break it open later in order to make new sense of his transaction with the situation. This becomes more difficult to do as the process continues. His choices become more committing, his moves more nearly irreversible. As the risk of uncertainty increases, so does the temptation to treat the view as the reality. Nevertheless, if the inquirer maintains his double-vision, even while deepening his commitment to a chosen frame, he increases his chances of arriving at a deeper and broader coherence of artifact and idea [p. 164].

For reasons examined more closely later, reading Schön, about three-quarters of the way through my year at State, at a time when I had already gained sufficient distance to reflect on my experience, dramatically reframed my earlier experiences of confusion and disillusionment. To put it simplistically yet honestly, Schön's validation of the inevitable uncertainties of professional practice and the continuing, if unacknowledged, process of thinking-while-doing helped me to forgive myself for my ineptitude and to reconsider what I was practicing in a more constructive light.

What sets Schön's epistemology apart from that implicit in the writings of interactive or interpersonalist clinical theorists such as Levenson (quoted earlier), is his central concern with how professionals learn. Not only does he decry the pitfalls of a professional's believing that with the right theory he or she can find the right answers, but he models, in painstaking detail, the purposeful yet often bumpy course that a "conversation with problematic materials" may take. Analyzing the transcripts of supervisory sessions, he identified "knowing" and "reflecting-in-action" in a way that made them accessible to me in my own struggles to determine what I knew, what I was doing, and what I hoped to accomplish as a psychotherapist. More specifically, Schön helped me to recognize that my experience of Kay was of the greatest importance to my learning and thinking about her.

Kay always "talked back." No matter what formulation or intervention I might hazard, she repeatedly surprised me. At our second encounter, for instance, two days after her black rage, she bubbled enthusiastically over a necklace I was wearing and came willingly to our first session. From larger than life, she shrank to about five foot two. This sort of unpredictability, a symptom of her disturbance, was also disturbing. Ultimately, however, I felt excited by, and in some ways admired, how stubborn and provocative this delinquent adolescent inpatient could be.

Chapter 2 traces as straightforwardly as possible the early history of my nine-month relationship with Kay. Organized roughly chronologically, it lays the groundwork for the reflections and revisions contained in the subsequent chapters. The history also introduces the other players in the drama: the unit as a whole, my treatment team (Team B), various representatives of other agencies, Kay's family, and others. By telling it like a story, I hope to evoke what it felt like to be an apprentice psychotherapist working with a demanding pa-

tient, within the complex system of State Hospital. Of equal importance, this narrative of often-confusing "facts" and characters emphasizes how badly I felt in need of a theory or technique to provide
direction for my efforts and definition for myself.

Chapters 3, 4, and 5 reprise and reexamine some of the events
presented in chapter 2 from three more theoretical perspectives that
I used to find my bearings. Ironically, none of the ideas I came to rely
on came from those interpersonalist theorists whom I so admired, a
fact that confused me at the time. Rather, I came to appreciate how
each point of view belonged to the growing repertoire of examples,
images, understandings, and actions by which I could begin to see
my unique relationship to Kay as something recognizable (Schön,
1983, p.138).

Indeed, nothing could differ more from an open-ended exploration of relational ambiguities than James Masterson's (1972) prescription for working with borderline adolescents, which I examine
in chapter 3. If anything, Masterson's clear, concise, and utterly
predictable clinical vignettes, strongly flavored with Margaret Mahler's developmental account of separation and individuation
(Mahler, Pine, and Bergman, 1975), reassured me that therapy had
an optimal course and I a well-defined task. As Schön's epistemology subsequently helped me to articulate, I needed to begin with
such a discipline if only to break it open later.

In fact, gravitating toward Masterson's theory was not even arbitrary. It was at first—and continued to be—a useful way to create
some order in the wild contradictions of Kay's complicated past and
to set forth three basic phases of treatment (testing, working
through, and separation), which were already familiar to the staff on
the unit. As daily interactions with Kay and the milieu eventually
made evident, however, I paid a price for assuming Masterson's
certainty. Increasingly, I experienced a gap between the calm objectivity of the therapist he portrayed and the unruliness of my own
emotions. His cursory identification of my reactions as countertransference only succeeded in making me ashamed.

Chapter 4 considers the murky but presently popular concept of
projective identification, which offered me a more tolerant view of
countertransference and enabled me to persist. Once again, however, when I rejected Masterson's conceptualization of the therapist's
role in favor of this friendlier notion, I could not justify my decision
in terms of a valued psychotherapeutic model. Rather, I picked up the

idea from various supervisors I respected, who described how it had helped them in similar cases. From Schön's point of view, they were demonstrating "reflection-in-action," a way of revising an original formulation to answer its unforeseen practical limitations. In other words, because Masterson's framework could no longer assimilate my experience in what it defined as the parameters of my work, I sought out a new way of making sense of it.

In a manner akin to what Erikson (1964) described as "disciplined subjectivity" (p. 53; see also Schön, 1983, pp. 116-118), projective identification offered me a way of interpreting my unanticipated reactions to my patient and suggested a strategy for using feelings to guide and evaluate our interactions. In doing so, it made a place within the therapy for what Schön labels "back talk." According to this new perspective, my therapeutic role was neither to suppress nor deny my personal involvement with Kay but, rather, to listen to what it might tell me about her inner life. Redefining my purpose as one of containing, tolerating, and digesting my patient's powerful emotions created a fresh problem-set with which I could move out from where I had earlier felt stuck.

As much as projective identification freed me to listen to the back talk within my relationship to Kay, however, it shut out the back talk from the milieu we were in. In chapter 5 I look at how I learned from the milieu literature yet another way of thinking about what I did. Introduced to me initially by McCaughan (1985), this point of view is most fully developed in Stanton and Schwartz's 1954 classic, *The Mental Hospital*. A milieu perspective helped me to view Kay's treatment as situated within a multidirectional framework; I gained a way of genuinely conversing with the other people with whom Kay and I worked.

My introduction to the milieu literature expanded dramatically my capacity to translate what Schön terms a "babble of voices" into meaningful dialogue with staff members about the significance of Kay's relationships with all of us. Equally important, by drawing on the complementary notions of parallel process and the split social field, I gained a useful distance from which to view interactions that had only upset me before. Already alert to the subtle and often wordless exchanges that can occur between an individual patient and therapist, I became aware of even more nuanced and many-layered communications within and between groups.

The interplay between thinking and doing engendered by my trial commitments to Masterson's theory and recommendations for treating borderline pathology, to the complex notion of projective identification, and to milieu therapy were most active and alive in approximately the same sequence as the chapters devoted to them. To a greater or lesser extent, they were embedded within a specific constellation of events and interactions and responsive to particular needs. It would be too neat and misleading, however, to say that one interpretative schema either "evolved into" or superseded the next. Even though my reflecting-in-action grew less arbitrary and more deeply and broadly coherent as my training progressed, I never fully abandoned any of these points of view. Rather, as I came increasingly to challenge my own quest for "right answers," I adopted a more ad hoc and, I believe, a more true-to-life way of proceeding. My training became unified, to use Schön's idiom, not by finding the best technique but by my activity as a "researcher in a practice context."

Running through and tying together the story of Kay's psychotherapy are my continuing reflections on what and how I learned from it. In my concluding chapter I address these issues more directly. Having abandoned the notion that I can straightforwardly apply theory to clinical practice, I recapitulate Schön's alternative method of inquiry in light of my experience. Drawing on Irwin Hoffman's (1983, 1990, 1991) development of a social-constructivist psychoanalytic paradigm, I also return to the notion of participant observation. Ironically (given how unavailable this stance seemed at the time), I think that this case demonstrates a viable sense of what it means to adopt such a therapeutic position. I then elaborate the specific ways that particular ideas and theories enhanced my participant observation of Kay by considering Lawrence Friedman's (1988) views in *The Anatomy of Psychotherapy*.

In writing this case study, I acknowledge the perhaps immodest intention of engaging my readers in a "conversation with indeterminate materials" similar to my own. A shared inspection of the underbelly of my learning can, I think, enhance our understanding of psychotherapeutic expertise and its acquisition and of how we might improve both. If it is true, as Schön suggested, that we can best exemplify the interplay of thinking and doing through case studies, whether written or presented, then their role in professional education deserves greater attention. Patrick Casement (1985), a British psychoanalyst who worked out a concept of "internal supervision" not unlike Schön's "reflection-in-action," made a similar argument for the significance of case studies when he observed that

> it is useful to use (or in Winnicott's sense, to "play with") clinical material outside the session. . . . Technique can be developed by taking time, away from the consulting room, for practicing with clinical material. Then, when in the presence of a patient, the process of internal supervision is more readily available when it is most needed [p. 39].

Because this case study draws from my first year of inpatient training, I do not offer it as an example of good—or even "good enough"—clinical practice. Instead, I offer an account of my own practicing that I hope will contribute to the practicing of others.

2

NOISY WORDS

When she was good she was very very good, and when
she was bad she was horrid.
Old English Nursery Rhyme

Kay once remarked matter-of-factly, but with an air of pride and sorrow, that she could make anyone believe anything. She was describing how the pimps of the "sex club" had beaten her for refusing to "play with herself" in front of a camera. When she arrived back at the group home, drunk and bleeding, she told the staff that a girl on the El had mugged her and they accepted her "cockama-mie" story. At the time, I expressed shock and outrage at the stupidity of these other caretakers. Since then, however, I have wondered if Kay was not commenting on my own gullibility, of which there were many instances over the course of the year. Alternately, she may have been complaining that I, like the pimp, forced her to expose herself in ways that threatened her self-esteem. Interpretations abound, some more plausible than others, but none with the reassuring solidity of fact.

In this chapter, accordingly, I present a collection of written por-traits—of Kay and myself and a host of others—shaded by ambigu-ities, deceptions, divided loyalties, and conflicting purposes, as much as they are illuminated by occasional moments of insight and

13

collaboration. As such, the content of the chapter differs from the more theoretical formulations of subsequent chapters in emphasis but not in kind. The specific theories I will discuss later—concerning the borderline patient, projective identification, and the milieu—are also ways of creating portraits, of putting together who someone is and the significance of what he or she does. What I learned in working with Kay, however, is the extent to which such characterizations are developed and revised in dynamic interplay—or, in Schön's view, "conversation"—with the stories others tell, not the least of which are the patient's own. The interpretations I voiced others either applauded or derided, qualified or contradicted, but they never left them unanswered. In the following pages, I want to convey what it was like to work amidst and respond to this "babble of voices" (Schön, 1983, p. 17) by surveying and commenting on what I and others wrote about Kay in reports, hospital charts, passalongs, and personal notes.

Because Kay's record is so voluminous, I have divided the chapter into two sections: in the first I attempt to pull together Kay's history prior to her coming to State; in the second I examine the early weeks of her hospitalization. These linked chronologies, separated neatly into before and after, do not represent, however, my actual experience in coming to know Kay. To begin with, I did not receive a reliable case history when she arrived or even a clear sense of why State admitted her. Instead, how I gathered and composed her fragmentary past interwove itself with the treatment. The past and the present inscribed themselves in one another.

What is more, the very ways in which I constructed Kay's elusive sense of self intermeshed closely with my sense of my own role. Paraphrasing an analogy from Margaret Mahler, I could describe Kay's treatment as our complementary processes of separation and individuation; the psychological birth was my own as much as hers. Gradually over the months, our reciprocal constructions of each other grew more stable as each of us grew more confident, she of herself as a "self" and I of myself as her psychotherapist. In this chapter the focus is on Kay; a more thorough discussion of the development of my own thinking will follow.

A BABBLE OF VOICES

Contradictions seemingly rooted in Kay's soul stretched back to before her birth and made gathering up her history a bewildering task. A passage from her probation officer's report, written in December 1985, demonstrates just how garbled the account could become. Referring to an interview with Kay's father, it reads as follows:

> He initially stated his childhood was a happy one, however, when the man was about 14 years of age his parents were fighting quite a bit and Mr. Z's father was drinking. Mr. Z was about 20 years of age when this occurred. And PO understands thru various resources [sic] that Mr. Z's father shot his mother to death during this argument.

Other versions of this extreme act of the family's violence are more coherent, but none offers so apt an introduction to the dizzying, breathtaking confusion that seeking to understand Kay's life could engender.

She was born on February 1, 1969, in California, within a year of her parents' marriage. Her father was in the Navy and away from home a lot; her mother was an alcoholic and also absent often. According to a social history provided by Mr. Z in September 1984, he stopped receiving letters from his wife when the baby was four months old; when he returned to California, he discovered that Mrs. Z had moved in with another man. A pattern of disappearances and reconciliations continued throughout the marriage, with Mrs. Z "running away" and Mr. Z finding her. A son, Joey, was born in 1972. In 1974 Mrs. Z left for the last time, her children in tow; Mr. Z did not follow. By then the family was in the Midwest, where Mr. Z was a truck driver. According to Mr. Z, after the separation, and divorce a year later, Mrs. Z and the children moved from one hotel to the next. Yet, as he explained it in 1984, he was reluctant to remove Kay and Joey from this "chaotic environment" because of the demands of his job. In any event, Mrs. Z soon returned to San Diego, where her mother and sister resided. She was apparently drinking heavily and was sexually promiscuous.

Kay boasted to me more than once that she had no need to keep "journals and diaries and stuff" because her memory was so sharp. She claimed she could remember the day she learned to walk, for instance, and the day Joey was born. Her recollections of "bad times" were especially vivid. Declaring that she was *born with problems*," she singled out as particularly difficult the time when she was 4 1/2 and her mother left her father. Less plausibly but more poignantly, she claimed to recall an incident of her parents' arguing years earlier; just a baby, she crawled between their legs and had her finger stepped on. Not surprisingly, the moral of many of her memories was that "the grown-ups let you down."

In 1978, when Kay was nine, her mother took the two children for a "visit" to their father and left them there. Kay's probation officer reported (again in 1985) that Mr. Z "seemed to be very surprised that the children were coming and indeed his present wife was surprised, as she did not know he had two children." He had been remarried for two years. The report continues:

> Both children were apparently quite damaged by then. . . . They had not been prepared that they were going to live permanently with their father [and they] had a great deal of difficulty accepting their step-mother. They were seen by Mr. Z and his new wife as well as the school authorities as generally undisciplined and hyperactive children who were not amenable to any controls. As time went on mother seemed to contact them by phone and kept them in a state of insecurity by continuing to promise them that they could return to California.

A story Kay told in 1984, interpreting a picture of a girl sitting with an older woman who is reading, suggests her own experience of her mother's desertion and the way she romanticized it to make it more bearable:

> There is this little girl. Her mother went away to Paris. Her mother is a famous model. She always stays at home. The housekeeper's trying to cheer her up by playing with her and reading to her. But it doesn't do any good. As time goes on she starts resenting her mother more and more each day and year. When she is 16, she just leaves and gets her own job. She and mother stay in touch, and mother finally understands what she did.

The ambiguity of her conclusion—does the mother finally understand her own actions or those of her daughter?—seems to highlight a confusion about just who is responsible and for what.

Kay portrayed her relationship with Joey both less ambivalently and more idealistically. He, like she, suffered the damage of inconsistent parents and, later on, of inconsistent—and ever-changing—child care workers. Brother and sister were allies, united in their distrust of—and longing for—caregiving adults. Joey also elicited a sort of maternal feeling in Kay: her baby brother needed and deserved her protection, she often declared; she had learned from the school of hard knocks and wanted to shield him from a similar fate. As she learned of Joey's eventual placement in foster and group homes, Kay responded angrily and even despairingly to their separation. She needed and clung to the conviction that someone else shared her life and loved her. The one time that they met in the hospital during Kay's sojourn at State, both she and Joey looked touchingly pleased and awkward, like a sister and brother.

The years between 1978 and 1982 were turbulent and ended with Mr. Z's second divorce and his signing over his custody of Kay to the Children's Aid Society (CAS). As recently as 1985 (the last time an interview with him is documented), Mr. Z persisted in blaming his daughter for the dissolution of his marriage. According to Kay, her father had been physically abusive not only to his children, but to his second wife, Nancy. In a telephone interview with Kay's State social worker in January 1986, Nancy confirmed the reported abuse and also her own past inability to take care of the children. During Kay's hospitalization Nancy asked at least twice to visit her, but the treatment team refused on clinical grounds. Nancy reported that she and her current live-in boyfriend were contemplating marriage and the eventual adoption of Joey.

Authorities first referred Kay to juvenile court on February 16, 1982, as an "ungovernable" runaway. Removed from her father's home on April 19, over the next 3 1/2 years she spent time in at least four psychiatric hospitals (including State), and the Children's Aid Society placed her, for varying lengths of time, in two group homes, a shelter, a foster home, two out-of-state therapeutic schools, and (twice) in the city's juvenile detention center euphemistically called the Juvenile Home. Kay had ten "station adjustments" for physically assaulting others, damaging property, thieving, drinking, and running away. She had already appeared in court eight times for these offenses before the police arrested her on August 8, 1984, for aggravated criminal sexual assault. Charged as an adult for the latter crime, she pleaded guilty in November 1985.

Together with her criminal identity as a child molester, Kay's past as a prostitute (while she lived in a group home) played a key role in how staff viewed her on the unit. Figuring out the actual dates of her prostitution, however, was almost impossible, in part due to her many moves and the conflicting reports spawned by her transience.

One report placed the prostitution as early as 1980; it is most likely, however, that it occurred between the summer of 1982 and the summer of 1983. The confusion was perpetuated, I think, by how emotionally charged an issue the "sex club" was. Kay herself alternately raged against and romanticized her life "on the street"; her CAS workers (who were legally responsible) seemed to vacillate between feeling guilt and resentment; and the unit staff probably felt disturbed that caretakers like themselves had exploited the sexuality of their 13-year-old charge.

Two radically different accounts of her father's response to her prostitution are especially illustrative of how others' needs and agendas could distort Kay's history. According to the 1984 social history provided by Mr. Z:

> When she ran away from the home [in the summer of 1983] . . . the people at [the home] reported that they could not locate Katharine. [Mr. Z] enlisted the help of his brothers and in one evening found Katharine. By this time he had learned of the existence of the sex club at the residence and he decided not to return her to their care. For three months she seemed to do fairly well with him but again ran away and was picked up by the police. This time, the Children's Aid Society placed her in a foster home on the south side. He had considerable concerns about a foster home, but felt the only alternative was to take her back home, which he was not prepared to do.

If not a hero in this version, Mr. Z at least appears involved in his daughter's life in a way that demonstrates concern and a realistic appraisal of his own limitations as a parent.

By contrast, Kay's probation officer wrote in 1985 (based largely on what Kay had told her) that Kay returned "voluntarily" to her father's home in September 1983 and pleaded that he allow her to stay, even though "this was the father, who the girl had stated, often had physically abused her in the past." The probation officer reported that after the court granted permission, with several provisos, there were no major difficulties for three months, but that in December the court's "Special Investigation Unit" interviewed Kay, having somehow established her participation in the prostitution ring:

> As a result the police officers came to the girl's home and interviewed her and the father became aware for the first time of the girl's sexual

adventures. He became very incensed with her behavior and the girl stated that in January the father actually "choked me," according to the information by the minor respondent to this PO. PO was aware that the father's method of parenting the minor respondent had always been very severe.

Kay, in the probation officer's account, emerges as a child whose crimes occurred because she had had caretakers who blamed her, instead of forgiving her, for what she could not help.

I only met Mr. Z twice, both times very briefly. To the best of my knowledge, no one at State ever spoke to him at any length, although the social worker made one attempt to interview him. (He failed to come in.) He visited Kay rarely and did not receive encouragement from any staff member to get more involved. By contrast, I got to know the probation officer rather well and considered her one of several de facto members of Kay's treatment team at the hospital. Her relative familiarity to me as well as Kay—and the fact that I liked her—contributed to my inclination to believe her version of events. Of greater importance, her story cast Kay into the role of a victim of circumstance and supported my need to see her as fundamentally innocent. While far too simple, this is the rendering of Kay with which I began.

Everyone agreed that Kay herself was an unreliable historian, a conclusion based largely on the tenuousness of her sense of self and the inconsistencies in her record. Interestingly, however, given my early constructions of her case, Kay rarely cast herself as a victim when discussing her prostitution. If anything, she flaunted how "good" she had been to her customers and how her body had been admired and desired. When she was angry, she would often declare her intention to return to hooking, where she knew others needed her and where she would make good money besides. More generally, Kay wanted me to see her as in control, as my notes from our session on October 24 make clear:[1]

---

[1] Here, as elsewhere, quotations are from my therapy notes and do not represent verbatim quotes from Kay herself. The notes were usually written within a day of her session, however, and provide a reasonably accurate account of what we said. While I have fleshed out my shorthand, I have left a sometimes confusing alternation between first- and third-person pronouns as I wrote it at the time. I think that the degree of ambiguity this conveys—of who is actually speaking about whom—is true to the frequently enmeshed quality of my interactions with my patient.

I mention the milieu meeting [where other patients talked about drinking and Kay reportedly offered some no-nonsense advice as an "hereditary alcoholic"]. She says she could tell them a lot (I under-score what she has to offer them). Even Tom, who's done a lot of drugs and stuff—she's probably more experienced. She's been in AA, Al-Anon, Alateen—and one other group. She'd done lots of drugs too. She was a heroin and cocaine addict while prostituting. No track marks (she shows me) because her mom's a nurse, so Kay knew what she was doing. Had $500-a-day habit; did more and more prostituting to support habit. She thinks of all the money she could've saved—*awful!* (Tries to calculate it—incomprehensible.) Went cold turkey at Juvenile Home; acted threatening so no one would know. Put in solitary where not able to come out. Sweated it out.

Coexisting with her insistence that she would be fine if only she could escape from "the system's" oppressiveness was Kay's equally strong need to see herself as "in charge" no matter what. She occasionally acknowledged the "brick wall" she had built up around herself as a consequence of having grown up in a violent and unpredictable world or the many masks she had donned to keep herself protected. At times, she laced these admissions with expres-sions of loneliness or regret; equally often, however, she was defiant or aloof. Above all else, Kay seemed to need to act even more outrageously than anything that anyone might tell about her. Through her own self-portrayals she defied anyone to understand her experience and strove to create herself as tough, street-smart, and able to "sweat it out."

After running away from her father in January 1984, Kay lived in the juvenile detention center, a shelter, another group home, and a foster placement, all within five months. Her alleged sexual abuse of two little girls (aged three and five) occurred in the foster home in July of that year. Given her dedication to reinterpreting, embellish-ing, and justifying her life, Kay's persistent refusal at State to speak directly about the abuse charges was all the more striking. Alert to the slightest opening, I asked her about the incident more than once, and each time she loudly denied that any wrongdoing had occurred. She accused me of trying to force her to talk and demanded to know if the judge had made discussion of the abuse a prerequisite for discharge. (As far as I knew he had not, and I told her so.) She was fully aware that she had pleaded guilty, but she insisted that this had been a pragmatic decision calculated to get her case transferred from adult to juvenile court and to avoid going to jail. She passion-ately declared her love for children and denied doing anything that could possibly hurt them.

Looking back, I am aware that my own needs and self-image contributed to my interpretation of this contradictory information. Rightly or wrongly, I was sensitive to Kay's accusations of forcing her to talk, and I regularly dropped my confrontations with her on the sexual abuse issue. My reasoning at the time was that issues of trust, manipulation, and coercion within the therapy were as important as getting Kay to open up about the criminal charges per se. I am better able to admit now how my desire to have her perceive me as a nice person may also have contributed to my reticence. What is more, *I* needed to like Kay, and without her open confession I could main-tain my hope that others had misrepresented or exaggerated the situation.

Knowing that Kay *had* "confessed" to her former psychiatrist, Dr. P, on the Adolescent Unit at University Hospital, which admitted her on August 29, 1984, made my position of willed ignorance more difficult to maintain. Dr. P's letter to CAS a month later provided the fullest account that I have of what allegedly occurred:

> It appears that two children in the house witnessed overt sexual activity on the part of their mother. As is common in such a circum-stance, these children then began to play sexual games and did this with Katharine. She reports two occasions in which this took place; in the first, which took place in mid-July [1984], the children apparently talked about doing with Katharine what they saw their mother doing with "Lonzo," an abbreviation of the mother's boyfriend's name. Katharine allowed this to go on and seemingly made no effort to stop it. On the second occasion two weeks later the children once again began to play, fondling her breast and licking her vagina. Once again, according to her statement, Katharine made no effort to stop the process.

Dr. P was convinced that Kay needed inpatient psychotherapy, and he wanted to treat her. His account of the abuse formed the centerpiece of his appeal to CAS to extend funding for a lengthy hospitalization. He interpreted to them, as he stated he had to Kay, that in abusing the children "she did the same thing toward [them] as had been done toward her." He noted that Kay understood this "intellectually," but had "no real awareness that her behavior with the children might be damaging to them." After a substantial discussion of Kay's past history and personality dynamics, Dr. P concluded:

> Although we are diffident in suggesting that she be left here, since after all we are paid, nevertheless she is beginning to make relationships here. To move her is only to repeat the trauma of her separations. We believe that any compromise of these recommendations will make for a failure of intervention. The risk with children such as Katharine is that when inadequate efforts to help are made, these fail and ultimately these children are labelled as bad and evil by society. They are then incarcerated in a variety of correctional settings and their prognosis is extremely unsatisfactory.

He requested—and received—six months to work with her, and then three more. Kay remained hospitalized at University for ten months in all.

Not surprisingly, given my similar desire to treat Kay as an inpatient, I felt attracted to Dr. P's formulation and adopted a version of it as my own in my discussions with Team B. I also referred to another event from the same month as the abuse—the murder of a close friend of Kay's, Maggie—to make a sympathetic case for what Kay had undergone.

Maggie was a resident of the group home where Kay had been a prostitute, although I do not know if she herself belonged to the "sex club." They had known each other for 2 1/2 years and, at least in retrospect, Kay both identified with and idealized her friend; she told me that Maggie was a "recovering alcoholic" like herself, calling her "the only person I believed in." Of the greatest importance, Maggie believed in Kay and would encourage her by saying, "Kid, you have only one life to live." No records that I have give any details of her murder. Kay, who never claimed to know either, concluded her version of Maggie's life with a melodramatic flourish that I thought belied her deeper feeling: "The good die young."

No written report or evaluation that I have links the trauma of Maggie's murder with Kay's sexual abuse of the little girls, making me wonder if my doing so served my own needs more than hers. I was moved—but was I also taken in?—by Kay's tearful testimonial to a lost friend. Perhaps the image of friendly intimacy between two young women appealed to me and mitigated and made more tolerable the charge of aggravated criminal sexual assault. In any event, hearing about Maggie was one of several moments that cemented my affection for Kay at a time when she was almost unremittingly obnoxious.

The suspicion that Kay was pulling the wool over my eyes never left me entirely. Although I felt increasingly more confident over the year that I could distill a more or less forthright communication from Kay's need to boast, posture, and manipulate, doubts lurked. Unfortunately, but not surprisingly, none of Kay's four psychological evaluations, completed between 1981 and 1985, clarified who Kay *really* was. Instead, they most frequently characterized her as ambivalent and, directly or indirectly, made it clear that she aroused similarly mixed feelings and impressions in others. The uncertainty amongst her caretakers had very real consequences for her treatment and long before the battles fought over her at State began, fundamentally similar disagreements about her problems and their solutions had already become established.

Sometimes I argued against myself; often I argued against others. Others had recorded similarly conflicted and conflictual opinions, which only added to my confusion. The chief psychiatrist at the Maryland placement where Kay had resided for two months just prior to coming to State, for instance, seemed a model of indecision when he wrote the following in his discharge summary:

> Katharine undoubtably [sic] sees her discharge from the [placement] as another "rejection" although at a conscious level, she herself is anxious to leave. In spite of her anxiety to leave, however, she is also ambivalent about leaving.

When opposing camps formed between caretakers—roughly, those who advocated punishment versus those who advocated help—the consequences were sometimes even more serious. I found an especially dramatic instance of this (from 1984) documented in the probation officer's 1985 report:

> It was while the girl was in the Juvenile Home in February and also part of March 1984, PO observed that the girl seemed distraught and upset. . . . Also, she verbalized a great desire to be placed in a psychiatric ward. She seemed to be truly distraught . . . The girl was inter-

viewed by several people . . . and it was felt that she did not deserve or
need the treatment of an intensive psychiatric ward or hospital, as she
had requested.

Only six months later, Dr. P stated that long-term hospitalization
was "indispensable."

Even at University, with Dr. P in charge of her care, controversies
continued. This is most evident in the inpatient progress notes that
Dr. C wrote about Kay whenever Dr. P was away. While I never spoke
to anyone at University and received only the public records of Kay's
treatment there, I could read staff dissension between the lines of Dr.
C's report of January 10, 1985:

> We also talked about why Dr. P likes her so much. It's very clear that
> she's very bad, but afterwards in terms of the psychotherapy, she has
> considerable insight in what's gone wrong. . . . I also discussed with
> her my concern about her being here when Dr. P returns. In some
> ways, her behavior is such from time to time that it is no longer
> tolerable because in the beginning when she was first here, Dr. P made
> allowances for her behavior because of what happened to her in the
> past and she had just entered the program. She has been long enough
> at this point [sic] to be held accountable for what she does rather than
> to be given excuses.

A week later, Dr. C apparently had sorted out his ambivalence to
some extent: "She is very likeable when she is working hard in her
treatment. Unfortunately, when I am not her therapist and Dr. P is
present, I see her as the staff do because her rages remain as horrible
as they ever were."

While Kay was at University she ran away twice; broke a staff
person's arm; and received trials of a variety of psychoactive drugs,
including Mellaril, Tofranil, and lithium. Dr. P twice banished her to
the Juvenile Home in order to "confront her with reality." Far more
disturbing than Kay's rages and how others responded to them,
though, was a more basic uncertainty about how long CAS would
continue to pay her bills. I do not know how long Dr. P wanted to
keep Kay hospitalized, but his notes implied to me that he thought
CAS was aborting his efforts. He felt his own commitment to the
case undermined in turn, and he wrote on March 11, 1985, "Arrangements are going to be made to transfer her fairly soon if CAS

will not be able to carry through with her until the end of her treatment."

In my first session with Kay, she angrily condemned CAS for barring her return to University. With no use for diplomacy or minced words, she said CAS would not pay for her treatment there. According to my notes, she went on to compare State very unfavorably to the much more prestigious University Hospital:

> If she had to go back to a hospital she wanted to go [to University]. But it doesn't do any good to talk. She had the "best therapist in the world" and it did no good—so why should she talk? She'd rather go to jail. . . . At least in jail she can *smoke*. At University there were rules about smoking too, but staff let you get around them because they knew they were "therapeutic". . . . She says at a certain point that the kids here are "crazy." When I point out that at University she was also on a psychiatric unit, she says she knows that, but that was a "program for adolescents." Have I seen some of the kids here?! I say that this too is a program for adolescents and she says she's just prejudiced: she liked University and she doesn't like it here.

My supervisor suggested to me that Kay's violent misconduct during the summer after her discharge from University may have been a ploy to get readmitted there. Certainly it had helped to convince two residential placements—one in Tennessee and the other in Maryland—that they could not keep her. For weeks I did not realize that Kay *had* been in two places, and I was not confident about what had happened until quite late in the year.

Kay, discharged from University on June 25, 1985, went to a placement in Tennessee highly recommended by Dr. P. Two CAS caseworkers accompanied her, not one as was customary in similar cases, although one of them, Kay informed me scornfully, was an alcoholic (she drank Jack Daniels in the hotel room). Within two weeks at this placement, according to Mrs. W, the director of the second one, Kay had "torn up" her room and her stereo. Placed in detention until they could arrange a transfer, CAS then had their charge flown to Maryland.

The discharge summary from Kay's Maryland placement that accompanied her to State began by emphasizing that while Kay was "tough," she was "nothing [the placement staff] couldn't handle." She aimed to shock—by piercing the hole in her nose, flaunting her

punk appearance and sordid past, and generally making herself out
to be somebody special. Despite all this, she was basically cooperative and gradually settled down. She had been taking lithium prior
to leaving University but refused to continue, saying she wanted to
control her "mood swings" on her own. The wrench in the works of
this relatively calm adjustment was a phone call from her mother on
September 13 or 14. Mrs. Z, then in a halfway house for alcoholics in
Minnesota, was due for discharge in February. The conversations
with her mother revived for Kay (as calls would again and again while
she was at State) an old and durable fantasy of living a "normal
family life" with her mother and younger brother, Joey. Kay's
behavior deteriorated rapidly and dramatically, and, on September
15, she physically threatened another resident. Because staff at the
placement were not ready to handle violence and Kay would not
comply with medication, they recommended her rehospitalization.
On the night before she left for State, she dyed her naturally blond
hair black.

I later learned that Kay's transfer had also been the consequence
of rivalries between CAS and the placement, in addition to the
disruption wreaked by her mother's phone call. (How her misconduct may have been, in part, a response to these disagreements I will
consider more fully in the chapter devoted to the milieu.) On
September 11, Mrs. W told me by phone in April, she had given CAS
an ultimatum: either assign Kay one case manager, or she would ask
her to leave. A specific argument precipitated Mrs. W's demand—in
contrast to CAS, she did not think Mrs. Z should contact her
daughter—but its significance was more general: who was to be in
charge of Kay's care? Because CAS did not comply with her wishes,
Mrs. W followed through on her threat. Kay arrived at State on
September 29th.

EARLY ARGUMENTS

Over the early months of Kay's hospitalization, my supervisor frequently complained that there was too much "noise" in my presentation of the case, by which he meant the plethora of conflicting
details that he felt distracted me from the psychotherapeutic task at
hand. I, meanwhile, bemoaned the episodic quality of my work and
my discomfiting inability to anticipate what might happen next.
Looking back, I think we were both responding to the difficulty of

maintaining our focus on a patient defined so inconsistently. Kay was an adolescent plagued either with too many selves or none at all. Her self-presentation, while dramatic, was typically contradictory, and this lack of self-definition made her—and me—vulnerable to others' assumptions about her.

Compounding the ambiguities of her ill-defined self was my own insecurity as a novice psychotherapist. Without much past experience with emotionally disturbed adolescents, perplexed by how best to proceed, I struggled to narrate intelligibly what I was doing, with whom, and why—a task made all the more difficult amidst the "babble of voices" that debated her care. Personal and institutional needs competed and often clashed with the goals of psychotherapy, forcing me to confront and to question whether and how I was practicing psychotherapy at all.

Ironically, but tellingly, Kay's hospital stay at State became dominated by her leaving. First of all, she ran away on November 1, just a month after her admission. Because her escape seemed to me and the staff to repudiate our skill and effort, her return two weeks later ignited heated debates about whether to keep her. Even when these arguments subsided and it became clear that Kay's hospitalization would continue, a recognition of the difficulties of eventually placing a 17-year-old delinquent then dominated the treatment. Given this unpredictability and the controversy Kay aroused, for the eight months after her running I worked under the shadow of her next unanticipated departure.

Even now I wonder if I should have spotted Kay's intention to run and tried to prevent it. Reading through the notes of her first month on the unit, I see hints of her plan everywhere. Yet I was not alone in feeling stunned by her disappearence. We all took it personally, as a judgment on our abilities to assess and manage delinquent characters and misconducts. Although Kay first came to State spitting and screaming, for instance, we understood this behavior as typical resistance and nothing to make a fuss about. Very few adolescents want to be hospitalized, and even fewer would admit it if they did. Kay, in fact, became fascinated from the start by an unusual patient who had been on the unit quite willingly for 1 1/2 years. As early as October 16, she marveled that a "*normal* kid" like Debbi "would not even be leaving this *year!*" The staff favored Debbi, the exception that proved the rule, as practically one of them. Threats and curses, like Kay's, were far more common from adolescent patients.

Still, Kay's anger, directed at me as vehemently as against anyone else, was distressing. Her angry rejection of the help I wanted to give her had no place in my early frame of reference as a psychotherapist. If anything, I had imagined my role as a beneficent godmother whose mission was to empathize and bequeath insight and understanding. Kay seemed to cast me in the role of evil witch instead. The more she perceived me as oppressive, the nicer I tried to become.

My self-image as a psychotherapist, coupled with the virulence of her temper, made me especially susceptible to Kay's incessant arguments that another hospitalization was unnecessary. I felt swayed by laments that she hadn't had a free moment to herself since July '84. "Nobody here is on my side, they don't know what my experience is [and] they're trying to change how I look," Kay complained, insisting that all she wanted was "a chance on the outside . . . to get out and go to a foster home and go to school and get a job." She devised one scheme after another to get her way: she would hire a lawyer and sue CAS; she would convince her father's brother to adopt her; she would so violate the "Big Four" rules (No Sex, No Drugs, No Aggression, No Running) that we would kick her out. She even intimated that she had "a trick up [her] sleeve to tell that judge."

Painfully uncertain of how to respond, I vacillated between tough and nice and felt at home with neither. On one hand, because I sympathized with her despair at being "screwed" by "the system," I accommodated all her moods and tried hard to answer her questions. On the other hand, however, for all my desire that she see me as one person who truly was on her side, I never really questioned her need to remain on the unit. At the time, this did not represent clinical acumen so much as my need to hang on to my first real patient.

My reaction to a request Kay made on October 16 illustrates the ambivalence I experienced about what to do and who to be. She wanted permission to give her portfolio to "someone who is connected to some hotshot in the art world [and to] store some stuff with this guy, like her summer things." In retrospect, it was evident that this transfer of her possessions was part of her escape scheme. This was the first any of us had heard of Kay's artistic ambitions, and even at the time I was skeptical of her extravagant predictions about her future as an artist and doubted seriously her art world connections. (In fact, she eventually demonstrated some drawing ability, but—as with most everything else—little discipline or consistent motivation.) Because I wanted to be the good guy, however, I submerged my suspicions and discussed her plan with her as if it were straightforward. My passalong from later the same day, filled with quotes, questions, and conflicting information, strongly suggests the mistrust I was unable to admit openly:

> Kay has asked to have a distant relative, "Joe," pick up her "portfolio" and some of her belongings. I referred her to [her social worker], but thought this would be OK—is it? In general, Kay continues to be extremely demanding and hostile in sessions. She did let slip how she wishes she could go home to her mother. Rita.

While staff exhibited far less of a need to make Kay happy, they too claimed not to see any difficulty with having the portfolio picked up, and they approved of the plan. I brought the good news to Kay like a gift.

My delight at the immediate improvement in Kay's mood again masked my doubts and prevented me from looking clearly at her unpredictability and volatility. On October 17, I allowed her to charm me by her talk of jewelry making, her love of animals, and her wish someday ("but not yet") to write the story of her life. When I asked about her high spirits, she reported joking with staff members about running away, an answer I recorded in my notes:

> Well, one thing that could've made me feel good [is that] staff took her to the laundry room, not just once, but *2* times! Plus, they'd had a good laugh about it because 3 staff had taken 4 kids—so in case she ran away 2 staff could go after her and one stay with the other kids—They told her about it afterwards. . . . It meant they were beginning to accept her (implication = trust her too). She'd been upset because at University they'd kept kids on the unit for 2 days, but she'd been here 3 *weeks*!

The reference to staff's (and perhaps her own) apprehensions about Kay running is there, but I chose not to respond to it. My particularly confusing use of pronouns in this note—did the trip to the laundry room make me or Kay feel good?—also suggests that my wish to feel positively about the treatment interfered with my achieving a more balanced view. I wanted to share my enthusiasm and not my uncertainties, as evidenced by my next passalong:

> Kay was feeling very good today. After half hour of talking about her art, jewelry-making, etc., she finally said that she was happy because staff took her to the laundry room *twice*—she feels like staff are beginning to trust her about running.

I do not recall more direct discussions of what the real risks of her running might be.

I did ask Kay at least once about her wishes to escape. She scoffed that that would be "stupid," adding, "as you very well know!" Besides, she pointed out with seeming practicality, she didn't "have enough money." At the same time, she was willing to admit, disarmingly, that while she was aware of her impulsivity, she could control it "just like that" (with a snap of her fingers). Whether the test of her self-control would be to take just one drink or to walk away calmly from an argument, she would be capable *as soon as we freed her*. Not really persuaded by her boastful claims, I nonetheless did not squarely confront how her actions belied them. With very little provocation she might fly off the handle, burst into tears, laugh uproariously, or grow icily silent. On the very day that she was feeling so good, in fact, she so lost her temper that staff had to place her in full leather restraints (FLRs).

In looking back, the biggest example of my vulnerability to deception—and self-deception—revolved around who would accompany Kay to court on November 1. The court had set this date for her to appear before the judge on the charges of sexually molesting the two little girls in 1984. Kay's lawyer, a highly competent young woman who worked for a legal aid society, had advised her to plead guilty at that time in order to get the charges reduced and the case transferred into juvenile court, and Kay had agreed to do so.

As the date approached, I felt distressed that Kay devoted far more of her attention to who would be at court than to her admission of guilt. She devoted most of her energy to arranging a luncheon, after the court appearence, with her CAS caseworker, whom she wanted to accompany her. Even though she could ridicule him cruelly for his "nervousness," she claimed pathetically that he was as close to family as she had and that she might never see him again as CAS had removed him from her case. Besides, she added dolefully, she deserved to have some kind of "pass" like the other kids on the unit. The treatment team felt otherwise and informed Kay on October 23 that a State worker would also go along. Stating that she was "angry—no upset," Kay worked to convince me that she would not run:

> We should know already that she won't run—she's told us she won't. "And you know, this program's not so bad." She feels as if she's been trying to settle in, getting to know people, etc., and it's as if it doesn't make any difference. . . . She feels like we don't trust her. . . . [Besides] they're people she's beginning to like and she doesn't want to disappoint them.

Remarkably, in light of subsequent events, Kay's concluding argument against State staff's accompanying her to court, according to my notes, was not wanting to "say good-bye." She implied, and I failed to question, that as soon as she pleaded guilty, the authorities would whisk her off to jail. Preoccupied with the sexual abuse per se and the need to discuss it, I interpreted this concern with good-byes as a fear of humiliation. As Kay soberly agreed, we stayed with that issue, and only later did I consider other reasons she might have to bid us farewell.

Kay did not limit her lobbying efforts against the staff's decision to me. Arguments rehearsed in our sessions—including her fears of appearing "nasty"—showed up in passalongs and nursing notes. Because I believed that who went with her was irrelevant to what was really going on, I gradually, if implicitly, came to take her side. Apparently, so did other team members, for reasons of their own, and at the October 30th Team B meeting we granted permission for her to go to court accompanied by only CAS. I delivered the news of this decision to Kay like a reward for her beginning to open up.

My satisfaction at identifying the "real issues" was short-lived, however. Immediate and vehement protests from Kay's lawyer ended in the permission being rescinded, luncheon plans being denied, and Kay's State social worker being assigned to go with her—with no consultation with me (it was my day off). I was furious. That Kay would be angry at me again was tiresome, but I felt that much more was at stake. By rights, I was in charge of her care, not her lawyer, I fumed; that the team apparently did not think so made me feel inconsequential. What was worse, now *I* felt humiliated in the eyes of my patient.

The social worker, possibly anticipating my wrath, informed me of the change in plans in a passalong rather than in person:

Rita, after conferring with Kay's lawyer [and other members of the treatment team] it was decided that I would accompany Kay on Friday because of the lunch-related concerns. Kay is upset and I have assured her that this happened without your knowledge. Kay should be ready at 9:00.

I did not acknowledge the merits of the new arrangements because I never seriously considered that Kay would run away. I was wrong.

According to the social worker's note in Kay's chart, both she and the CAS caseworker accompanied Kay to court on November 1. Since Kay had pleaded guilty as planned, the court lessened the charge and transferred the case from adult to juvenile court. However, instead of agreeing to return immediately to the hospital, as they had planned, Kay persuaded her chaperones to let her visit her former unit. The note continued:

Katharine had taken two pieces of artwork and a portfolio with her. She dropped those off at University Hospital. She gave them to a staff member to give them to Emily. . . . After court and after stopping at University Hospital, Mr. B (driving), K (in the front seat), and I (in back seat) were returning to State. At Huron and State, K got out of the car as the light turned green and ran.

My own shocked dismay notwithstanding, I comforted myself with the recognition that I was not alone in being fooled.

This slender solace did not prevent me from blaming myself for what had happened; it seemed a judgment on my competence. Others—including several patients who had kept Kay's confidences to themselves—also felt guilty. I did not believe the nurse supervisor when she reassured me that runaways usually came back, and I had even less confidence that the city police would succeed in tracking Kay down.

Thus, I again felt surprised when close to midnight on November 14 I received an excited phone call from the psychology intern on night duty, who trained on my unit. She had just readmitted Kay who was "okay," but "depressed." Together, the two had smoked a cigarette and chatted. Kay told the intern that she had been staying with her boyfriend. The boyfriend really loved her, she continued, and had grown increasingly alarmed at her expressions of despair. Finally, she had allowed him to call the police and they had brought her in. The conversation sounded sweet and sad, and I felt grateful to the intern for telling me so quickly.

We only felt the full effect of Kay's running when she returned. Everyone was angry. Kay herself lashed out with characteristic contrariness and denied everything she had told the intern. Far from depressed, she had been ecstatically happy, she said, having gotten a job, an apartment, and a puppy who needed her. She had had wonderful sex and now thought she was pregnant; this too was good news, as a baby would be someone who would love her absolutely. She ridiculed our concerns that she might commit suicide; she had not wanted to die and had lied just to avoid going to jail. (She was smart, she explained, and knew that suicidal kids go to the hospital while runaways go to prison.) Now that she was back on the unit, though, she had once again changed her mind. She hated the program and adamantly stated that she would refuse to comply. On and on she went, her strident, mocking voice provoking and answering the crescendo of arguments about her.

While everyone's feelings about Kay were mixed to some extent, her treatment team debated three basic formulations or diagnoses: sociopathic, borderline, or essentially normal. If either the first or the last, the arguments went, she did not belong with us on a psychiatric unit; while normal individuals do not *need* help from a hospital, sociopathic ones will refuse it and never get better. If Kay's pathology destined her to a marginal existence of survival, no matter what others gave her, some on the treatment team held, the hospital had a duty to discharge her and give her bed to someone who could use it. When I argued that Kay was depressed, others insisted she was manipulative; when I proposed that she was borderline, others countered that criminal would be more accurate.

Both in Team B meetings and at the nurses' station, I clung tenaciously to my belief that Kay needed long-term help for her emotional disturbance. Yet in spite of my scorn for those who thought State should discharge Kay, I too had grave doubts about how best to respond to her, engendered both by my own anger and a wish not to appear ridiculous.

Anger and the threat of humiliation went frequently together. In my notes from our second session after her return, for instance, I barely concealed my cold fury at Kay, which was compounded by my awareness of the paper-thin walls of the office that broadcast her insults to me all over the unit. I told her, amongst other things, that

she had "messed up" her treatment planning and observed omi-
nously that I did not know if she would remain at the hospital; the
detention center seemed likely. Kay, in turn, accused me, amongst
other things, of being "withholding," with some justification. In the
early weeks of her treatment, I was certainly unable to be forthcoming with her about what I was feeling. With a mixture of embarrassed confusion and diffidence, I wrote the following to the staff in
that afternoon's passalong:

> As most of the unit overheard, Kay was extremely angry during
> session, demanding I answer her questions about her discharge date/
> planning, but then unable to hear what I said. I identified this as a
> problem, but she refused to work on it. Rightly or wrongly, I let her
> know that if she cannot work out in our program she may have to
> return [to the juvenile detention center]. Although this is in fact true,
> I'm aware of my own anger . . . Rita.

Kay was certainly aware of the controversy swirling about her and
had her own opinions of how others should see her. In her psychotherapy session on January 24, for example, she asked me where we
would send her if we decided she was "not treatable." By this, she
meant "not capable of making progress" and "not getting involved."
In her case, she insisted, the issue was not capability, but desire; she
wanted neither treatment nor involvement—but still she was curious. When she mentioned a specific placement, a therapeutic school
where a friend of hers lived, I asked her what she imagined it was
like; I recorded our exchange in my notes:

> She imagines it's kind of like State. (A pause.) The school might be
> better. (And how would you be if you went there?) Quiet at first, until
> she got to know people. She'd resent being there. (Kind of like here?)
> Yeah. (How does she think that staff see her here?) As a stubborn,
> willful child. (But you were wondering about "untreatable"; do you
> know why you thought of that now?) No - a long silence. (Where did
> you go?) I was thinking of a tattoo I'm going to get, I'm not sure
> where . . .

Kay's abrupt shift to tattooing only demonstrated her self-
assessment: she was a stubborn, willful child who used her body to
shield her inner confusion and distract the eye of the beholder. She

wanted me to believe that she would do whatever and answer whomever she wanted.

As the debate about her escalated, the treatment team leader proposed an extraordinary intervention: we would invite Kay to join us on December 4 and contribute to the decisions we were making about her future. We would clearly and concisely present her with her options and with a timetable: either she must comply consistently with the program before her next court date, December 20th, or State would tell the judge that she could not benefit from further treatment. Presumably, at that point CAS would transfer her somewhere else. The nurse supervisor, a very powerful presence on the unit, endorsed the suggestion. Thus, despite my grave, if poorly articulated, misgivings, the team agreed to the plan.

Typically, patients received weekly feedback from their teams on how they were doing, but the rationale was always to bolster the structure that the teams were providing. Our offering Kay, instead, the choice of whether or not to continue flew in the face of the unit's policy that the professional staff was in charge. Reflecting the far more usual approach was a message Kay herself received on November 25: "When staff feel that you no longer need hospitalization you will be discharged. Staff run your treatment plan, not you." I worried that we were contradicting ourselves and thereby undermining our authority.

Although I wanted consistency, for myself as much as for Kay, I was, as I wrote in my personal notes in anticipation of the meeting, "not optimistic about [her] staying. I think she's so eager to make her *own* decision—to have some sense of self-control—that she'll decide to leave." Indeed, two days prior to the meeting, Kay signed a "five-day," a legal document requiring the hospital to release a patient within five business days unless a judge mandates continued inpatient care. Even though this was a common act of rebellion on the unit, I was so sensitive to her defiance and its reception, that my interpretation was one-sided. Only later, in light of subsequent developments, did I consider that Kay might have been hoping that we would hold her back.

The December 4 meeting ushered in the unhappiest month of my training at the hospital. Convinced that others did not respect my assessment of Kay's needs and potential, and even more sure that I would lose her, I felt ineffectual and unsupported. Even worse, I saw my taking a stand with the team as confirmation of my hypocrisy. I did not agree with the ultimatum, but I acted as if I did. The meeting itself went as planned, lasting about one half-hour. Kay was initially contemptuous of the options we presented her, but then ended up in tears.

My pessimism notwithstanding, the special meeting proved a turning point both for Kay and me. For her especially, its effects were immediate and constructive. Within hours of the conference she had re-dyed her hair to its natural blond color, helping us somehow to notice that she no longer wore a nose-ring. Later that evening she spoke tearfully to a milieu worker about "resigning" herself to the program; while this resignation was erratic, it attested to a significant change of heart.

The meeting's positive influence on me was less direct and forthcoming, and I had to wait until a two-week Christmas holiday to gain enough distance to appreciate it. Simply put, it took this low point in my training to force me to get more help. As Kay's treatment had grown more complicated, I had felt increasingly stymied by my State supervisor's admonitions to "turn down the noise." I did not think that I could, nor was I persuaded that details of Kay's past and both her and my present on-unit relationships to the team were irrelevant to the therapy. I determined to seek outside supervision from my adviser who had worked at State for several years, was continuing to supervise interns there, and had influenced my decision to train there. Rather than simply discuss case material, we agreed to a reading course on psychoanalytically informed hospital-based treatment. What we read ultimately had a directly beneficial effect, as I discuss in depth in Chapter 5.

My request for help did not reap exclusively positive rewards, though. While it certainly bolstered my flagging sense of being able to think and act for myself, I used my reading course to avoid dealing directly with my unhappiness with my State supervisor, a senior clinician and assistant unit chief on A-1. I now can identify at least two major sources of tension between us. First, our personal styles differed dramatically: I freely—perhaps too freely—expressed my anxieties and preoccupations whereas my supervisor had a more laconic manner. I sometimes imagined that I overwhelmed him with the loose ends (the "noise") that I myself could not tie together. I felt torn between my wish to do well in his eyes and my growing resentment at not feeling understood and supported. Second, I ultimately found the milieu or systemic approach introduced to me by my advisor far more helpful than the more dyadic approach advocated by my State supervisor. I simply could not "turn down the noise" of the multiple relationships the therapy entailed until I had a greater appreciation of their relevance for and influence on the help I was trying to provide. Regrettably, however, my supervisor and I never attained sufficient perspective on the system we both participated in to discuss our differences in depth, and for quite some time I covertly devalued what he—and other State clinicians—could offer me while idealizing my "outside" teacher. In Chapter 4 I examine more specifically how this repudiation of my supervisor (and the team) had detrimental effects on the treatment.

Over time, though, I gradually began to learn new ways to conceptualize my role and practice that helped me to identify what I was doing and discuss it more constructively—and less antagonistically—with my supervisor and team members. While a full examination of these new and more self-conscious approaches forms the subject of the following chapters, let me conclude this one with the two hypotheses about the effects of the December 4 team meeting with Kay that I held at the time.

My first hypothesis stemmed from my eventual recognition that the unit at State was not unique in its treatment plans or its ultimatums to Kay. For all the institutions involved, in fact, the conference that I considered so unusual was just one in a series. Less than a week after the special meeting, to give an instance, Kay was visited by her probation officer. With the full authority of the criminal justice system to back her up, she told Kay unambiguously and forcefully to count on being in one "locked facility" or another *at least* until she was 18. If she signed a "five-day," she would go to jail; it was as simple as that.

The judge himself was even more authoritative, as I learned the three times that I met him. Particularly at my first court appearance, on December 20—when her social worker, probation officer, CAS worker, two lawyers, and I accompanied Kay—his influence was impressive. A paternalistic, perceptive, and fundamentally sympathetic man, he presented a stern exterior to all of us and tolerated few ambiguities and no disagreement. Perhaps if I had been more confident in my position, I would have resented his self-assurance. As it was, his command reassured and bolstered me as much as it sobered my patient.

My first hypothesis explained Kay's improvement—and the hospital's contribution to it—in terms of the far more extensive and powerful legal system to which we all answered. My second hypothesis identified the change as illusory, a playing out of just another one of Kay's many personae. This latter speculation grew out of my reflections, in January and February, on Kay's frequent discussions of her life as a prostitute. As about most things in her past, she felt conflicted about what she had done: while she had hated the coercion of the pimps, she had taken pride in "being good." Her mixed feelings about State, I soon decided, followed a similar pattern, which I interpreted thus: Kay resented her forced compliance in the program, but would nonetheless deliver what the customer (therapist) required.

With each of these hypotheses about the parameters of the treatment, I believed, for a time, that I had discovered *the* explanation for how the special meeting had made a difference in Kay's behavior. Either she was responding to the external threats of the criminal courts—quite apart from what we did—or she was responding to the internal compulsions of her own long-ingrained habits. Only later, as I became more knowledgeable and self-aware as a psychotherapist could I articulate my own positive influence on Kay's improvement as integral to a complex system of personalities and relationships.

In this chapter I have tried to demonstrate through a variety of stories told by and about Kay how difficult her "self" was to get to know and how unsettling its ambiguities were to experience. In the chapters that follow I describe several ways in which I tried to clarify and come to terms with what it meant to work with Kay. In doing so, I reprise and reexamine stories already told, and they will shift in their importance. Beginning with the literature on borderline patients and moving on to a consideration of projective identification and milieu therapy, I will, in a sense, tell stories about the main story: how I used theories to construct and interpret the situations in which I was engaged.

3

CONFLICTING WORDS

She fakes, just like a woman,
And she takes, just like a woman,
She makes love, just like a woman,
But she breaks just like a little girl.
Bob Dylan, "Just Like a Woman"

In the previous chapter I attempted to convey the confusing variety of stories told about Kay, both prior to and following her admission to State. The early weeks of her treatment there were characterized by debates, often angry—with her but especially amongst ourselves—about "who" she was, as if we all felt an urgent need to establish her identity once and for all. In many respects, Erikson's (1956) concept of identity diffusion aptly summarizes the indeterminacy of Kay's character. It also informs much of the literature on so-called borderline adolescents and was a theoretical perspective toward which I turned initially in my efforts to construct both my case and my role as a psychotherapist.[1] How I used this theory,

---

[1] Pulling together a composite sketch of adolescent patients diagnosed as borderline, Erikson (1956) stated that "they all suffer from *acute identity diffusion*, a (temporary or final) inability of their egos to establish an identity" (p. 239). Otto Kernberg (1978a) echoed Erikson when he wrote, "I cannot stress sufficiently that the most fundamental aspect of the diagnosis of borderline personality organization involves the evaluation of the presence or absence of the syndrome of identity diffusion" (p. 317).

rhetorically as well as conceptually, throughout the year, is the subject of this chapter.

In this, as well as the chapters on projective identification and milieu therapy, I will not provide an exhaustive literature review. Innumerable surveys of the borderline literature already exist (e.g., Sugerman and Lerner, 1980; Vela, Gottlieb, and Gottlieb, 1983; and M. Stone, 1986), many of which agree that a unifying concept of the disorder is impossible to attain (Pine's 1974 and 1983 analyses of the borderline diagnosis for children are particularly trenchant). Rather, I will concentrate primarily on the work of James Masterson (1972, 1975, 1980), addressed specifically to the intensive inpatient treatment of borderline adolescents.[2]

I came across Masterson's work somewhat by chance, although the popularity of the borderline concept and Masterson's relative fame as a theorist make my discovery unremarkable. Masterson's son and I attended the same professional school, and early in my studies there his father came to speak. The lecture room was packed with students, teachers, and professionals from throughout the city. A sense of collective excitement conferred respect upon the speaker even before he opened his mouth. When he did, he spoke clearly and compellingly of borderline concepts, handing out diagrammatic representations of "part objects" and "whole objects" and liberally illustrating his meaning with case material. More generally, my teachers and supervisors often cited Masterson's work with Donald Rinsley (1975; see also Rinsley, 1982) as clinically helpful, especially in the context of hospital treatment.

Let me emphasize at the outset, though, that with Masterson's ideas, as with the others I consider in later chapters, my aim is not to present how I applied theory to the "solution" of the case. Instead, the discussion of my particular use of Masterson exemplifies how theory helped me to begin "conversing" with radically "indeterminate materials," thereby initiating the ongoing process of "making sense of an uncertain situation that initially [made] no sense" (Schön, 1983, p. 40).

This chapter divides into two sections. In the first I start by giving an overview of Masterson's theory and psychotherapeutic tech-

---

[2] Even a cursory view of the recent literature makes evident the extent to which Masterson's views developed in collaboration with other theorists, most notably, Otto Kernberg, Donald Rinsley, and, especially, Margaret Mahler, whose conceptualization of the infant's "psychological birth" I elaborate later in this chapter.

nique, paying close attention to his own constructions of clinical materials. I discuss the extent to which the theory provided a plausible account of Kay's personal and interpersonal difficulties and a strategy for plotting her hospital course. Despite its indisputable usefulness, however, this definition of who Kay was proved limited and, in important respects, untherapeutic. In the second section of this chapter I describe my increasing dissatisfaction with the understanding of Kay's treatment that Masterson's position suggested in an attempt to conceptualize what was at the time an experience of growing disjunction between the therapeutic ideal that he modeled and my practicing as it actually occurred.

THE BORDERLINE ADOLESCENT'S STORY

For all its pretensions to objectivity and scientific rigor, Margaret Mahler's (Mahler et al., 1975) depiction of the toddler's achievement of separation and individuation has an almost visceral immediateness. Each time I read her descriptions of Wendy, Sam, or Bruce in *The Psychological Birth of the Human Infant*, I can feel their exhilaration as they learn to walk, rushing out to greet a world that, for a brief time, seems theirs to explore and delight in. More poignantly, Mahler also evokes that moment of truth when children at this stage recognize the world's dangerous hugeness and the irrevocable distance their steps have placed between them and the safety of their mother's arms. Thus ushered in is the rocky rapprochement subphase of our original struggle for a sense of self, a crisis of profound ambivalence in which the drive for independence and autonomy regularly counters our emotional dependence on mother:

> Conflicts ensued that seemed to hinge upon the desire to be separate, grand, and omnipotent, on the one hand, and to have mother magically fulfill their wishes, without their having to recognize that help was actually coming from the outside, on the other [p. 95].

The vicissitudes of this crucial period of human development, within the context of the relationship with mother, animate James Masterson's conceptualization of the borderline adolescent. He opened his 1972 book, *Treatment of the Borderline Adolescent*, with the assertion that if a mother is emotionally unwilling or unable to encourage her toddler's increasing independence and is at the same time intolerant of the child's ambivalence and unavailable as a safe harbor, "this tie that binds changes a normal developmental experience into one so fraught with intense feelings of abandonment that the child experiences it as a real rendezvous with death" (p. ix). Along the same lines, Mahler (1975) commented that

> the less emotionally available the mother is at the time of rapprochement, the more insistently and even desperately does the toddler attempt to woo her. In some cases, this process drains so much of the child's available developmental energy that, as a result, not enough energy, not enough libido, and not enough constructive (neutralized) aggression are left for the evolution of the many ascending functions of the ego [p. 80].

Most important, according to both authors, such an unavailable mother denies the child the opportunity to resolve his or her ambivalence. As a result, children fail to achieve an emotional object constancy, the ability to integrate good and bad experiences into realistic representations of their mother and themselves. Their emotional experience, tied to the immediate, thus is overly dependent on the pleasurable or frustrating tenor of the moment. Through the mechanism of "splitting," the world becomes unstably divided into all-good and all-bad "part objects."

Equally serious disruptions in behavior complement the borderline's experiential discontinuities. Because "he is unable to evoke the image of the person when he is not present . . . he cannot mourn. Any object loss or separation becomes a disastrous calamity" (Masterson, 1972, p. 31). As borderlines encounter the stress of a renewed drive toward individuation in adolescence, they respond to the increasing pressure of abandonment fears with defensive rage and delinquency.

Drawing on these observational and theoretical underpinnings, Masterson elaborated a prescriptive agenda for the psychotherapeutic treatment of these troubled adolescents. From a series of case vignettes, he distilled a typical developmental narrative and plotted the characteristic stages of the therapeutic process. *Every* borderline child, he began, has a borderline mother who is intolerant of his or her drive toward independence and a father who is weak-willed and aloof. Given these family and developmental dynamics, by adolescence *every* borderline expresses depression, anger, fear, guilt, helplessness, and emptiness (which Masterson terms the "six psychiatric horsemen of the Apocalypse") in a range of inarticulate, antisocial, and/or self-destructive behaviors. In contrast to the parents, the psychotherapist must unambiguously and consistently interpret such conduct as a "desperate cry for help." Such help can best—and perhaps only—come from a long-term inpatient hospital setting where firm rules and regulations force adolescents to contain their impulsivity. They must acknowledge and work through the painful feelings that they have for so long tried to avoid.

Like the child described by Bettelheim (1975) who insisted on the same fairy tale being read to him over and over again, I relied on the sameness of Masterson's narratives to comfort myself that what seemed chaotic others had sorted out before. Even though his plot structures are formulaic and thus intellectually uninteresting, their very redundancy was reassuring. A note I wrote in Kay's chart, on January 20 summarizing the themes of the previous week's sessions illustrates the extent to which I used Masterson's descriptions as a pattern for sorting through and simplifying Kay's contradictory self-presentations and rapidly shifting emotions:

> Pt [patient] continues to circle around "her past," continually bringing it up. Her reaction to opening up and acknowledging how much she cared about what we thought of her . . . was first to retreat to her stance as a pseudo-mature adolescent and then, when the anxiety became overwhelming, she discharged by getting very angry. By the end of the week pt seemed sobered and more able to get in touch with her depression. As we discussed the difficulty she has observing her own feeling states pt began to cry, stating that she was afraid she couldn't do what we expected of her. Characteristically, it was hard for her to stay with this sense of inadequacy and she quickly retreated to saying she didn't *choose* to observe herself. In my assessment, pt's pattern of disclosure, withdrawal, anger, depression, disclosure is fairly typical of the borderline adolescent.

In Masterson's view, Kay's typical pattern of psychotherapeutic advance and retreat was not cause for discouragement but, rather, a reenactment of her original ambivalence within her relationship to her mother. My task, from his perspective, was to tolerate her virulent anger and flagrant misconduct while unrelentingly identifying and confronting her with interpretations of what they meant.

My use of Masterson's version of the borderline diagnosis was

simplistic, but far from arbitrary. Faced with the necessity of diag-
nosing Kay today, I would almost certainly use it again. In the
remainder of this section of the chapter, I focus on three aspects of
Masterson's theory to justify this decision. First, Kay's long-
troubled relationship with her mother, and especially her persistent
fantasies of a reunion that would right all wrongs, was consistent
with Masterson's developmental account of similar adolescents.
Second, and even more evident, the symptoms of her disturbance—
her impulsivity, delinquency, sexual promiscuity, and fluctuating
interpersonal ties—were, in his view, fundamental to the diagnosis.
Finally, what Masterson describes as the psychotherapeutic stages
of the adolescent's hospital course—testing, working through, and
separation—were useful in thinking about treatment goals and the
purposes of my interventions at various points during the year.

Everything about Mrs. Z suggested her unavailability to her
daughter. Most dramatic were the repeated, actual abandonments
Kay endured from her fourth month on; that her mother was an
alcoholic and also, apparently, sexually promiscuous only added to
my impression of her inadequacy as a parent. Although there is little
to suggest that she actively fostered her daughter's dependence, her
emotional and actual absences may well have diverted the toddler
from her developmental path as she struggled to gain and hold her
mother's attention.

A dream Kay had about her surrogate caretakers at State powerfully evoked the child's sense of desperation and what Masterson
called her "rendezvous with death." During the very early hours of
December 26, when she should have been asleep, a milieu worker
discovered Kay reading in her room. After first angrily cursing the
staff person for insisting she turn off the light, Kay later apologized.
The chart note continues:

> Said she was afraid to sleep as she has had bad dreams the past two
> nights. In one, she dreamt that she was in FLRs [full leather restraints]
> and her appendix burst and she screamed for staff, who finally came,
> saw the blood coming from her mouth, looked at her and left.

I never discussed this dream directly with Kay since I was myself
unavailable to her at the time, happily away from the hospital for a
two-week vacation. Whether or not my own withdrawal echoed that
of her mother, Kay's dream seems to represent graphically a young

child's sense of utter helplessness when her cries go unheeded. The image of being held in restraints is especially vivid: like the emotionally abandoned toddler, Kay, in her imaginative world, was crippled in her ability to stride forth self-confidently as an autonomous individual.

A similar sense of abandonment and a life-threatening loss of control infused a memory Kay revealed on February 13. My notes from the session begin as follows:

> [Kay] tells me that there'd been a fire alarm and that she'd gotten very scared because it reminded her of a fire when she and her brother almost died of smoke inhalation. Mother was smoking a cigarette, fell asleep, fire. Kids were in room, couldn't get out. Kay can't remember but thinks she and Joey jumped out of second-story window.

The representation of being trapped and suffocating is again suggestive of how Kay's experience of her mother's neglect, like the fire it caused, prohibited her natural exit from their originally symbiotic relationship. Because she was "asleep," the mother could not hear her children's shouts. With direct communication thus made impossible, there was no other recourse for the children but to take risky action.

Although she never visited while Kay was at State (despite numerous plans to do so), Mrs. Z telephoned frequently enough to fuel Kay's fantasies of their future life together and yet erratically enough to fuel her anger and despair. As described in the previous chapter, one such phone call, to Kay's previous placement, apparently triggered a deterioration in Kay's behavior serious enough to necessitate her rehospitalization.

At least four of the five times Kay actually needed full leather restraints while at State followed conversations with one of her parents. The ambivalence and behavioral disruption aroused by her inability to count on their promises to reform and care for her were evident in a letter Kay wrote to her father shortly after being removed from restraints on October 17. My notes from the next day's session read, in part:

> She reads a four page letter which is basically a clearly stated request/plea that her father acknowledge and do something about his contribution to her problems, as *she* is doing; that he begin to tear

down the brick wall he's built up around himself, as *she* is. She loves
him as a father, but hates him for what he's done to her and Joey·
. . . Tells me that if her father won't work on his problems then she'll
never get rid of hers because he caused so many of her problems that
she can't change if he won't.

Similarly, following another episode of being in restraints on February 9, Kay oscillated dramatically in her conversation with me
from cheerful chitchat, to heated anger, to tears. According to my
notes:

> Throughout the session I connect her anger and disappointment to
> her mother's not being reliable and coming through for her. [Kay]
> develops this by saying that even when her mother was physically
> present [Kay] couldn't tell if [mother] would be *with* her. Mother has no
> "maternal instinct," etc. Slips back frequently to blaming/anger at
> [unit] staff.

Mrs. Z's own difficulties in recognizing her daughter as an individual other than her "baby" became touchingly evident when (on
December 9) she sent Kay a 2 1/2-foot stuffed red hippo that she had
made and clothed in Kay's baby clothes and shoes. Kay's response
was complicated and tumultuous: initially thrilled, by noon she was
again infuriated at "the system," and by her afternoon therapy
session she was in tears. Mrs. Z's gift and Kay's response to it are at
least consistent with Masterson's hypothesis that the borderline's
mother clings to her child because of her own abandonment fears,
placing her child in an impossible bind. Kay herself may have gained
some awareness of (and thus distance from) this dilemma when,
several months later, she remarked ruefully that her mother had
been "shocked" that her daughter needed a size 36B bra. As Kay put
it, "she [hadn't] seen her children grow up."
    Closely related to Kay's longing to be mothered was her fre-
quently stated wish to have a baby of her own. Her fantasy seemed to
be of an exclusive and all-absorbing union; she imagined a child
utterly devoted and dependent on her. According to Masterson,
painful feelings of emptiness are intrinsic to the borderline's abandonment depression, and one can interpret pregnancy (as well as
drug and alcohol abuse) as the adolescent girl's efforts to "fill herself
up." Accompanying their hopes and fears are borderlines' somatic

preoccupations, anxious concerns that they have suffered physical, rather than emotional, damage.

In the weeks following her return to the hospital after running away, Kay was convinced that because she had had sex, she was certainly pregnant. She denied the physical evidence that she was not (menstruation) and insisted that she had a "medical problem." According to a nursing note documenting one such discussion:

> Graphically described her boyfriend and stated he may have knocked something around inside her, she may have appendix problem, or alluding to she may be having a miscarriage. Could not hear or accept that she may not have been pregnant. Complained about severe pains on her right side.

In this and similar instances, Kay experienced her emotional hurts and desires as physical realities. Rather than recognize her psychic incompleteness, she masked it with bodily concerns.[3]

Masterson's framework enabled me to fill in Kay's past history and present psychological states while helping me to find a way to engage and remain sensitive to my patient. Just as urgently, however, I needed to establish her treatability in the eyes of the team. For this, Masterson's descriptive symptomatology of the borderline diagnosis and overview of the adolescent's typical hospital course provided an essential supplement to my more speculative assumptions about Kay's subjective experience. Repulsed by her challenges and denigrations of my interpretations, I relied upon Masterson's (1972) claim that "the key to diagnosis is not the subjective symptoms which the patient will report, but his acting out behavior which is obvious to all" (p. 42) to guide my responses to her and my discussions with my team-mates.

"Acting out," as Masterson uses it, is a broad concept pulling together a wide range of multiply determined maladaptive behaviors. Aggressive acting out, as opposed to passive-agressive or obsessive-compulsive acting out, is most characteristic of the bor-

---

[3] Ironically, toward the end of her hospitalization, the results of a Pap smear established that Kay was suffering from "moderate dysplasia," precancerous cells of the cervix. Kay told me that the gynecologist who treated her confirmed her suspicion that her precocious sexual activity may have predisposed her to this condition. Her *psychological* response to being "damaged" I consider from a Kleinian perspective in chapter 4.

derline adolescent and includes a variety of antisocial behaviors, such as stealing, abusing drugs and alcohol, being sexually promiscuous, running away, and consorting with undesirable companions. Such conduct, according to Masterson (1972), is primarily "a defense against feeling depressed and remembering the desperation, abandonment, and helplessness associated with the pain of separation from the parent" (p. 43). He concluded, therefore, that "the more depressed the patient becomes the angrier he becomes" (p. 59).

Masterson's assumption that the borderlines' angry acting out can directly correlate with the extent of their depression was useful both for making sense of (if not accepting) Kay's past criminal behavior and for understanding and tolerating her concerted attacks against us. As described in the previous chapter, her history was replete with aggressive acting out, and her tough, "don't-mess-with-me" demeanor continued at the hospital. Cushioning the full brunt of her hostility for me, however, was my expectation that when we had successfully contained her impulsivity within the unit structure, the acting out would give way to an articulation of the pain underneath.[4]

A second, and closely related, source of Kay's defensive rage, according to Masterson's model, was the many ego defects she suffered as a result of her stunted emotional development. These defects included her impulsivity, low frustration tolerance, and tendency to distort her perceptions of reality. On the unit Kay's readiness to explode the minute she did not get her way, her narcissistic need to see herself as the smartest and sexiest, and her persistent and unrealistic fantasies of fame, revenge, and a "normal family life," all seemed attributable to a poorly consolidated sense of self.

Intrapsychic splitting, in many ways the hallmark of the borderline's psychic functioning, exemplifies the confluence of defensive-

---

[4] Unfortunately, my own empathy with her pain and minimization of the motivational force of her anger may well have seriously misled me in the first month of Kay's treatment. On the eve of her running away, for instance, I concluded a chart note by speculating that her depression was "deep-seated" and that her "feelings of abandonment [were] related to [her] low self-esteem and feelings of despair." Although I continue to believe that Kay was profoundly distressed, I hope that I would not be so quick now to discount the real possibility that continued acting out, even within the hospital, is very likely to occur.

ness and ego weaknesses. Not only are the patients unable to integrate the good and bad qualities of a significant other into a stable representation but they use this developmental defect to preserve their all-good image of their mother. Displacing their own aggressive hostility toward the mother onto an all-bad object, they are able to deny any conscious awareness of their mother's emotional desertion of them.

Kay's frequent raging against "the system"—and all of us within it—seemed the most obvious evidence of her defensive use of splitting and projection. Her conviction that her difficulties were all our fault effectively spared her parents any blame and left open the possibility of an eventual reunion with them. A passalong that I wrote in early April gives an especially vivid example of how any recognition of her parents' failings could ignite Kay's fury against everyone else:

> Kay is very upset about her mother's imminent discharge from the halfway house and move to her own apartment. Mother also talked to Kay about wanting to get custody of her brother (but not of her). Kay certainly got in touch with how hurt and rejected she feels. . . . But she also wanted to believe that State/the System could force her parents to take responsibility for her. It gave me new insight into why she hates State so much—and why she *needs* to hate us, to protect her (fading) hope that someday her parents will acknowledge their mistakes and make some of it up to her.

Finally, according to Masterson, the already hospitalized adolescent acts out to test the consistency of the hospital milieu and treatment staff. Far from rejecting psychotherapeutic interventions, borderlines push up against them to reassure themselves that the limits are clear and firm. The unit's clearly defined rules and regulations, as well as the staff's persistent efforts, in contrast to the past inconsistencies of their parents, eventually convince borderlines that staff are genuinely concerned about their welfare. Given this dynamic, during the first "testing" phase of the hospitalization the therapist's primary goal is to control the misconduct, thereby communicating his or her reliability to the patient. In Masterson's (1972) words:

> The basic job of management is to set limits in order to control the patient's acting out; to convert the patient from an actor and non-feeler

to a feeler and a talker, that is, at another level to interrupt his defenses against mourning so that the separation process can proceed and repair can be accomplished; and at a third and final level to establish the psychotherapist's competence and trustworthiness [p. 114].

If staff does not maintain such consistency on the unit, Masterson warned, the adolescent will feel provoked to "the same disappointment and rage that was provoked by his parents" (p. 116).

Masterson's way of saying who borderline adolescents were and how therapists should treat them was attractive because it promised to clean up an otherwise messy situation. I used his theory to exchange the indeterminacy of Kay's "identity diffusion" for the certainty of her diagnosis and to chart clearly the course her hospitalization (optimally) should take. Above all else, Masterson (1972) seemed to portray the therapist as indisputably in control, something I desperately wanted to be. In his case vignettes, he always sounded assured and decisive, and his interventions were superbly coordinated with those of the staff. Accordingly, he could assert that "the treatment is a process, a continuous series of changes, one laying the groundwork for and flowing into the other in a natural and logical manner—smooth transition from one phase to the next depends on the appropriate therapeutic procedure" (p. 109). I gravitated toward this benign, paternalistic figure whom I read as assuring me that he had the right answers; I admired his self-confidence and modeled formulations of my work along the narrative lines he provided.

Ultimately, however, this same paternalistic quality, which led me to base my interpretations and conception of my therapeutic role on his theory, became a stumbling block for my continued adherence to Masterson's point of view. The shift was gradual and, for some time, largely unrecognized. Writing my notes as if I was certain of what I knew and did, I used them to hide from myself (as well as others) how insecure I really felt. When such self-deception was no longer possible, I realized—to my dismay—that I had more in common with Masterson's patient than with his portrayal of the psychotherapist. However disturbed, the patient at least had an emotional life; the ideal therapist that I had constructed stayed impossibly calm, cool, and collected.

In concluding this chapter, I will elaborate on my discomfort with my earlier embrace of Masterson's paternalistic attitude and bring to light what I consider to be its hidden premises and implications. I will argue that in a variety of ways, I drew upon Masterson's theory to advocate, in effect, that therapists split their own object representations into the all-good (the therapist) and the all-bad (the borderline adolescent). In other words, I relied upon key theoretical distinctions to deny therapists' continuing issues with separation and individuation in their ill-fated attempt to recover for themselves what Mahler (1975) called "the forever lost illusion of omnipotence" (p. 222).[5]

CHALLENGING AUTHORITY

In a therapy session on February 28, Kay angrily wanted to know if I expected her to "*cry* all the time in session," if this was what I meant by her "doing work." Earlier in the day I had accompanied her, for the second time, to appear before the judge, and in large part she was attacking me because my assessment of her hospital course was not as rosy as her own. Even so, her question brought me face-to-face with my preference for her sadness over either her anger (which I found unsettling) or her many enthusiasms (which I dismissed as resistance).

Over time, this and other instances of Kay's "talking back" forced me to examine my own defensive use of Masterson's prescriptive agenda for treating the borderline adolescent. Eventually, I had to concede that Kay was not a helpless victim of fate, as I had come to believe, but, instead, an active participant in our ongoing interactions. I did not articulate many of my criticisms until much later; none of them prevented me from continuing to use Masterson's constructions. As with other theoretical perspectives with which I "conversed" throughout the year, however, my understanding of how and why I was using Masterson *did* change, informed by my continuing reflections on my relationship with Kay.

In contrast to Schön's conceptualization of a practitioner's "reflection-in-action," Masterson's theory has no way of accounting for the validity of a patient's "back talk." Instead, it assumes a medical

---

[5] Given the strong personal reasons I had first to embrace Masterson's views and then to repudiate them, I must acknowledge the possibility that what I identify as a critique of his theory is actually a critique of my use of his theory. In what follows I try to the best of my ability to maintain a distinction, although I do not think that one can ever fully divorce a theory from how it is put to use. As interesting—and relevant—an issue as this raises, it will need to await another essay for further exploration.

model of mental illness; Masterson conceived of the borderline adolescent as diseased and in need of the therapist's cure; proper diagnosis once made, the therapist could then logically administer appropriate—and clearly defined—procedures much as a physician would prescribe a drug or surgery for a physical ailment.

Borrowing an analogy from the study of infectious disease, Masterson (1972) contended that "each Borderline parent is a contagious agent carrying within himself the seeds that will spread the disorder to yet another generation" (p. 89). Elsewhere, in a characterization of his work with adolescents and their families, he broadened the analogy to include the therapist as a healer whose technical expertise is the key to the patient's recovery:

> One could compare the underlying family symbiosis to a boil or "abscess" that has caused drastic limitation of communication in the family to avoid the pain of separation-individuation. . . . The therapist, the most objective person in the group, is the only one who can guide the family to the center of the problem. When he does reach the "abscess" and lays bare the symbiosis and depression, the family reexperiences their original pain and suffering. The resulting emotional catharsis drains the "abscess," relieves the anxiety and depression and frees the family to repair the damage [pp. 16-17].

Masterson's analogies are notable for the almost perfect symmetry that they create between patient and therapist. Beginning with a fundamental polarization between sickness and health, one can generate a list of opposites that clearly differentiates the roles patient and therapist play. The patient's passivity, impulsivity, emotionality, and childishness contrast precisely with the therapist's activity, purposefulness, objectivity, and maturity. Inadvertently, I think, I took a small but crucial step from this dichotomization of descriptive qualities to a moral judgment that the patient is "bad" and his or her therapist "good." For a time, I used Masterson to paint as black and white the otherwise distressingly ambiguous relationship I had with Kay.

Because Masterson located the etiology of the borderline syndrome so squarely within the mother-child relationship, I did not immediately discern the susceptibility of his views to a conceptual splitting of patient and therapist into bad and good poles. I at first assumed that he theorized within an interactional framework, understanding both the child's and the mother's experience and be-havior in terms of mutually defined interpersonal roles. Whereas Masterson clearly described the therapist's influence on the patient, he scarcely mentioned how therapists themselves are reciprocally affected. Instead, a reenactment of the pathological symbiosis of the "infected" child's original relationship neatly opposes the profes-sional's objective—and "healthy"—detachment.

Even in his brief discussion of countertransference in *The Treat-ment of the Borderline Adolescent*, Masterson (1972) sharply cur-tailed the role of the therapist's subjectivity.[6] He admitted that in the face of "the most intense and most fundamental [feelings] in the human vernacular," it is "little wonder" that the therapist may be "upset" (p. 233). His ensuing examples make evident, however, that he considers such experiences to interfere with and even threaten the successful outcome of the treatment. He noted that counter-transference blocks are a particular problem for therapists with unresolved unconscious conflicts from earlier periods in their lives. For obvious reasons, I was most interested in his comment that such difficulties are not at all uncommon in trainees.

Masterson (1972) attributed a young psychotherapist's counter-transference to his or her own recent emergence from adolescent conflicts and to the correspondingly "fragile equilibrium" of the still-forming ego structure: "Confrontation with the mercurial emotions of his adolescent patients actually mobilizes his own latent conflicts, unresolved dependency needs and difficulties with tolerating hostil-ity. The therapist responds with his characteristic defenses" (p. 234).

Up to this point, I think Masterson's interpretations are plausible, although somewhat condescending to trainees. They suggest that, at least for novice therapists, a hidden subtext of the treatment is their identification with their patients in terms of their own concerns about dependence and autonomy. In his claim that the accom-plished therapist has learned "to contain the conflict within himself and allow as little as possible to affect his behavior with his patient," (1972, p. 233), though, Masterson implies that beginning therapists can realistically strive to remain unaffected by their patients as a

---

[6] More recently, Masterson (1983) published *Countertransference and Psychothera-peutic Technique*. Clearly responding to a demand that he address himself more fully to the therapist's subjective experience, these transcripts of supervisory sessions with psychotherapists-in-training are not much more than illustrations of his earlier claims.

goal of their training.[7] In other words, Masterson's formulation easily—and ironically—falls prey to the same defensive dynamic that he maintained is fundamental to the borderline's psychopathology. His use of absolute distinctions supports (albeit without explicitly endorsing) the assumption that therapists either are or should be immune to their patient's "disease." To the extent that I endorsed this assumption, I conferred upon therapists almost magical powers, not unlike the toddler who believes that he is "separate, grand, and omnipotent" and in no need of "help . . . coming from the outside" (Mahler et al., p. 96).[8]

Regrettably, my reliance, for a time, on Masterson's concepts to justify a definition of my psychotherapeutic role adversely affected how I negotiated my relationships with patients and colleagues alike. By using Masterson's theory to divorce what distinguished my identity as a therapist from my patient's characteristics, I effectively concluded that the borderline adolescent is incapable of reality-based judgments and emotions, irrespective of the specific context in which these occur. Whatever Kay said or did, moreover, I could interpret as meaning its opposite, even though Masterson provided no criteria for ascertaining when such translations were justified. Thus, for example, Kay's treatment team routinely, even automatically, interpreted her anger as part of her illness; we paid far too little attention to those situations in which it was perfectly appropriate. Let me illustrate what I mean.

Kay was frequently angry at CAS and the unit for the difficulties we seemed to have in coordinating our efforts. Even when meeting times were set weeks in advance, it was quite common to have them changed up to the last minute. A chart note from Kay's social worker describes one such occasion:

---

[7] In "The Patient as Interpreter of the Analyst's Experience," Irwin Hoffman (1983) offers an alternative view. He argues that "the analyst in the analytic situation is continuously having some sort of personal affective reaction that is a response to the patient's manner of relating to him. What is more, every patient knows that he is influencing the analyst's experience and that the freedom the analyst has to resist this influence is limited" (p. 411). The importance of Hoffman's "social paradigm" for psychoanalytic theory and practice, as well as its relevance for Schön's concept of "reflecting-in-action," I discuss more fully in my concluding chapter.

[8] Mahler herself, to whom Masterson owes so large a debt, is less sanguine. Reflecting on the personal motivations for her life's work, she observes that "a *lifelong, albeit diminishing emotional dependence on the mother is a universal truth of human existence*" (Mahler et al., 1975, p. 197; italics added).

> Kay was very angry because she had expected CAS to hold a case review on 2/19 and that will be delayed a week. She overreacts to anything which could be made to appear that "her workers do not have their act together." I am concerned that she says she wants to prepare for independent living but she continues to try to find someone to "adopt" her and loses control when a fantasy dissolves.

Because there are no details of how she expressed her anger, it is not possible to assess whether and how Kay was overreacting. What interests me, however, is the note's failure to recognize her legitimate reasons for being disappointed. The meeting had been arranged to discuss what treatment—and possible placement—recommendations to make when Kay appeared in court on February 28. Her wanting us to "have our act together" and to have a preview of what we were going to say to the judge does not, at least in retrospect, seem so out of line. Instead of granting her a right to be angry, however, the note goes on to express skepticism about her capacity for independence. The social worker apparently assumed that her present temper was, as always, a response to being confronted with her unreasonable "fantasies."

A treatment summary that I wrote about a week later gives a less obvious, but perhaps more insidious, example of how I drew upon Masterson's formulations to disavow any reality basis—and thus personal responsibility—for my patient's subjective state:

> Over the past two weeks the patient has been increasingly anxious about her treatment plan, the possibility of discharge planning, and her progress review in court on 2/28. . . . Given the patient's history of abandonment, which she now sets up to be repeated over and over again, coupled with her defensive need to appear pseudomature, one can only imagine the intensity of her apprehension. Along with this, the patient alternates between experiencing her therapist as a trustworthy ally and as a traitor, another caretaker who has let her down. Particularly since the patient learned she does not have a definite discharge plan she has focused much of her anger and disappointment onto the therapist. Interspersed with this preoccupation—and reliving of her old trauma—the patient has been able to make some connections with her present feelings and her familial relationships.

Although in this note I at least began by locating Kay's anxiety in the context of her actual situation, I immediately shifted my focus to her (presumably intrapsychic and pathological) "setting up" of her re-peated abandonment crises. With this established, I could then frame Kay's ambivalence toward me as if it were *only* a function of her internal dynamics. Further shielding myself from the discomfort of looking at my own contribution to her distress, I then interpreted her present feelings as straightforward repetitions of her feelings in the past.

My problem with the sort of formulation exemplified here is not that it is all wrong but that it is one-sided. I have no doubt that Kay did wrestle with ghosts from her childhood and that these colored her perceptions and disrupted her emotions. I am also persuaded that her improved equanimity as her hospitalization progressed depended, in part, on her identifying, interpreting, and laying to rest these old demons. The danger, however, of my overly defensive use of Masterson was that at the same time that I was insisting that *Kay* make these connections I was myself failing to appreciate the subtleties of my *own* connection to her.

Ostensibly, psychotherapy with the borderline adolescent aims to promote the patient's separation and individuation, including his or her capacity for autonomous choices and plans of action and partic-ipation in mutually respectful and satisfying interpersonal relation-ships. Because Masterson's theory does not offer positive definitions of what these capacities entail, however (both patient and therapist being defined negatively, as what the other is not), these treatment goals can all too easily become sabotaged. Particularly if therapists tacitly assume that the patient's feelings and conduct are *by defini-tion* unrealistic and irrational, they will be unable to respond appro-priately and specifically to what the patient says and does. Thus, much like the mother who cannot applaud her toddler's growing independence from her, these therapists inadvertently contribute to their patients' continued dependence on them.

In addition to denigrating Kay's capacities and blocking my ears to her "back talk," I also found in Masterson's theory a rationaliza-tion for my antipathy toward the staff. My initial response to Kay's running away is a case in point. According to Masterson, this kind of "acting out" could have had one of two motivations: either Kay was defending herself against the pain of attachment (and corre-sponding fears of loss), or she was reacting to the inconsistencies that she perceived in her care. Since I felt convinced that Kay needed long-term hospitalization, I freely blamed the staff for their apparent reluctance to treat her and thus for the discrepancies in how we conceptualized her care. This perspective alleviated my trouble-some worry that perhaps *I* was at fault. Not only were staff not heeding Kay's "desperate cry for help" (as I was), but, I believed, they were exacerbating her acting out by their failure to respond.

Looking back, I think that my own need for consistency over the first three months of Kay's hospitalization was as least as strong as hers (albeit unacknowledged). Ill-prepared to think either of short-term interventions, or of more extended treatment plans coordinated between several individuals or even institutions, I relied on Masterson's model to bolster my case for Kay's long-term treatment with *me*. She needed to know unambiguously, I argued, that I was in charge of her care at the hospital; the ongoing disagreements within the treatment team would only undermine this goal.[9]

Given the increasing severity of my criticisms of Masterson's formulations over the year—for not making room for Kay's and the staff's plausible commentary on the treatment or for their real and often powerful effects on me—I should give some consideration as to why and how I continued to use them. Briefly put, I think that Masterson's theory initiated me into a way of talking—about "acting out," "splitting," "testing," and "setting limits"— that had long been common parlance amongst the staff on the unit. Thus, at a practical level of interpersonal exchange, it provided a lingua franca for our discussions of the case. By (increasingly consciously) adopting a language established long before I arrived, I could begin to affiliate myself with my colleagues in our shared work with Kay. My growing appreciation for the fundamental necessity for teamwork recast my understanding of how I could use Masterson's theory (I address this more extensively in chapter 5, "Shared Words").

In this chapter I have examined how James Masterson's theory of the so-called borderline adolescent provided me with a lens for seeing through Kay's acting out, and an ideal blueprint on which to model my interventions. I have tried to show, as well, how in response to her "talking back" I came to challenge the assumptions that Masterson's conceptualizations implied. As I hope I have made obvious, I exaggerated what I consider legitimate criticisms out of a

---

[9] Kay's previous psychiatrist, working within a similar idiom, had made a comparable argument, as I was well aware, when he wrote CAS that "to move [Kay] is only to repeat the trauma of her separations."

need to conceptualize my persistent doubts and turmoil in a way that avoided concluding that I was seriously lacking as a therapist. The position that had initially bolstered my self-definition came to haunt it: I simply could not live up to an ideal of myself as calm, cool, and collected.

Following the dialectical course of my "learning-in-action," in the next chapter I look at alternate formulations for the phenomenon of countertransference, which, for a time, seemed to capture more accurately my experience with Kay. I turned from Masterson's views to the notion of projective identification, with which I could more readily integrate my own emotions into the aims of my work.[10]

---

[10] Countertransference, recast as an integral component to the therapeutic relationship and process, has become an increasingly popular idea in recent years. Tansey and Burke (1989) provide a lucid historical review of the varying definitions of the concept before advancing an intersubjective perspective that differs fundamentally from Masterson's. The concept of projective identification served as my introduction to such an alternate view.

4

MAGIC WORDS

I cannot overemphasize the enormously treatment-
facilitating value, as well as the comforting and liberating
value for the therapist personally, of locating where this or
that tormenting or otherwise upsetting countertransference
reaction links up with the patient's heretofore unconscious
and unclarified transference reactions to him.

Harold Searles,
"The Countertransference with the Borderline Patient"

On December 16, a month after Kay's return from running away from the hospital, I presented her case to an outside consultant who specialized in the psychotherapeutic treatment of juvenile sex offenders. At this conference, attended by most of my teammates, fellow students, and the milieu staff, I remarked,

> The first thing to know about Kay is the extent to which she arouses strong and often conflicting responses in others. I have found myself, in quick succession, alarmed, repulsed, moved, amused, infuriated, and above all *confused* by her. What I struggle with, in a funny way, is where *my* experience ends and where *hers* begins. I certainly don't want to deny my own countertransference, but it seems possible that— through something like "projective identification"—Kay is "communicating" through the powerful feelings she evokes or "puts into" me.

Projective identification was a new way of organizing my thinking about Kay, one that promised to solve the problem of my "interfering" emotions. Not only did the concept address how upset I had been, but it enabled me to recast my distress in a far more positive light.

This chapter describes and reflects upon my use of the concept of projective identification during what proved to be the most difficult period of Kay's hospitalization. In many respects, this concept provided an antidote to Masterson's minimization of the therapist's emotional involvement with his patients. While Masterson exudes certainty, projective identification embraces ambiguity; in contrast to Masterson's prescriptive and clearly ordered views on therapeutic interventions, projective identification tolerates the "horrible bloody mish-mash" of working with such severely disturbed individuals (Segal, 1974, p.57). Projective identification made my troubling feelings, which Masterson discounted or failed to mention at all, central to the psychotherapeutic task. In sum, by shifting from Masterson to this alternative perspective, I could acknowledge and talk about my experience as intrinsic to, not hindering, my interactions with Kay.

Despite my having studied it poorly and come up with an idiosyncratic interpretation, projective identification left a lasting and essentially fortuitous impression on my formulation of the case. In the first section of this chapter, I define how I understood it and recapitulate the personal and interpersonal contingencies (described more fully in Chapter 1) that led me to use it. Following this, in the next section, I illustrate and reflect on the ways in which the concept modified my appreciation of my role as a psychotherapist and, in turn, my actual interactions with Kay. As helpful as projective identification indisputably was, however, it shielded me from dealing directly with the unit and my supervisor in ways that were ultimately detrimental. I examine the reasons for this in concluding the chapter.

RESCUED FROM UNRESOLVED CONFLICTS

At the time when I relied most heavily on projective identification, I had read not a word of the extensive literature about it. Instead, it was something in the air, a bit of folklore picked up from various supervisors who had also struggled with disturbing patients and for whom the concept had seemed to work. From the start, in other words, projective identification was a practical notion, as much a part of my situation as it was a strategy for gaining some distance from it. I had not studied it systematically and then applied it in the field; rather, it seemed embedded in the case, awaiting my discovery. Miraculously there when I needed it to transform my experience, projective identification's emergence at times had a magical quality.

Having read at least some of the literature since, I find Thomas Ogden's formulation of projective identification to be most similar to what my supervisors handed on to me, and I will use that version here and elsewhere in this chapter as a backdrop for my more ad hoc adaptation of the term.[1] In *Projective Identification and Psychotherapeutic Technique* Ogden (1982) began by defining projective identification as

> a concept that addresses the way in which feeling-states corresponding to the unconscious fantasies of one person (the projector) are engendered in and processed by another person (the recipient), that is, the way in which one person makes use of another person to experience and contain an aspect of himself. The projector has the primarily unconscious fantasy of getting rid of an unwanted or endangered part of himself (including internal objects) and of depositing that part in a powerfully controlling way [p. 1].

This "getting rid of an unwanted or endangered part" of the self seemed to me to be similar to what Masterson called splitting, whereby borderline adolescents, unable to hold together in their mind's eye the contradictory qualities of persons, act as if others were either all-good or all-bad. By focusing on what it feels like to be the recipient of such attributions, the concept of projective identification redefined what had been intrapsychic and made it an interpersonal phenomenon.

More than with most psychological constructs, grasping the sense of this frequently mystifying exchange of feelings and fantasies

---

[1] Whereas I think that Masterson's theory—and not just my use of it—warrants the sort of critique I have provided, I am in no way impugning Thomas Ogden's work in my criticisms of projective identification. As I have stated, I read his book on the concept well after my training at State and find it far and away the clearest and most sensible presentation of this complex notion.

depends on being able to ground it in an actual experience. Good clinical use of it can occur only if the therapist has immediate access to how his or her emotional state finely tunes into the patient's. Accordingly, Ogden (1982) wrote:

> Projective identification is a clinical-level conceptualization with three phenomenological referents, all of which lie entirely within the realm of observable psychological and interpersonal experience: (1) the projector's unconscious fantasies (observable through their derivatives, such as associations, dreams, parapraxes, and so forth); (2) forms of interpersonal pressure that are often subtle, but verifiable; and (3) countertransference (a real, yet underutilized source of analyzable data) [p. 9].

Not incidentally, his insistence on its phenomenological basis enabled Ogden to distance projective identification from Melanie Klein, who coined it (1946, 1955). Obviously unable to refuse her her place in the idea's history, he argued that, as presently conceived, projective identification owes no allegiance to any one theory. (I discuss this claim further in the third section of this chapter.)

According to Wilfred Bion (1959, 1967), a Kleinian analyst whose views Ogden found more acceptable, therapists serve as a "container" for their patients' disavowed feelings. Much like a mother bird, the therapist "digests" and makes more palatable emotions that were initially too powerful or threatening and then "feeds" them back in a form that the patient can more easily assimilate. Perhaps because I was myself so needy, metaphors of holding and feeding were particularly attractive to me. What fascinated me most, however, was the tantalizing possibility that feelings that *I* was experiencing were not wholly my own.

Immediately prior to my discovery of projective identification— scarcely a month after Kay had run away from State—I was disturbed by a desire to run away myself. While she was gone I had felt guilty, as if I had been responsible; when she returned, I felt unsupported in my attempts to carry on. After weeks of anxiety about my capacities as a therapist and team player, I realized with a shock that I wanted to get out. This craving was worse than feeling alone and discouraged; while unpleasant, the latter were easily compatible with my sense of the arduousness of my work. A wish to escape, instead, was enormously threatening to my self-definition. If not a good therapist, I was at least responsible and persistent, surely it meant something awful about my character if I wanted to give up.

Projective identification gave me a way to resolve this dilemma, an idea I tentatively proposed at the December 16 case conference. If Kay had put into me her own desperate wishes to escape, then I could interpret my feelings as a communication from her. Because of her need to appear tough and self-sufficient, she was unable simply to tell me how out of control she felt. Instead, she unconsciously fantasized depositing her vulnerabilities into me in a way that powerfully controlled my own experience. Thus, far from being a source of shame or interference, I could tap my subjectivity as a valuable source of empathic understanding. As Ogden (1982) reassuringly put it:

> These feelings are not necessarily a reflection of unmanageable pathology on the part of the therapist. The capacity to allow oneself to be vulnerable to experiencing one's anxieties, conflicts, and fears is one facet of what is meant by being open to serving as a container for the patient's projective identifications [p. 117].

What is more, because I was better able than Kay to contain such painful affect, I could help her process and reintegrate what she had disowned about herself. In short, projective identification created a new space for my practicing that mitigated, by reinterpreting, my temptation to run away.

In some respects, my reinterpretation of Kay's indirect, nonverbal communication resembled Masterson's argument that the therapist must hear—through or behind his or her overt rage and misconduct—the borderline adolescent's "desperate cry for help." For Masterson, however, therapists' ability to hear depends on their being relatively unencumbered by their own personal reactions to their patients' behavior. Asserting the importance of the phenomenon of projective identification, Ogden instead maintained that it is these personal reactions themselves that provide essential clues to what the patient is communicating:

> Countertransference analysis is the means by which the therapist attempts to understand and make therapeutic use of his response to the patient. This is not an effort to "get through," "filter out," or "overcome" what the therapist recognizes as a reflection of his own

> personality. Rather, the therapist makes use of his self-understanding
> to determine how his feelings and thoughts have been uniquely
> shaped and colored by his present experience with his patient at this
> point in the therapy and in particular by the specific qualities of the
> patient's predominant transferences to the therapist [pp. 72-73].

This alternative conceptualization of countertransference legiti-
mized my emotional involvement with Kay in a way Masterson's had
not.

At the same time, however, my adaptation of projective identification in this instance was less evenhanded than Ogden's and,
ironically, fostered a more subtle form of running away. Unspeak-
ably relieved that my subversive feelings originated with Kay and
not myself, I allowed myself to believe that they really had nothing
to do with me at all. Ogden, by contrast, insisted that projective
identification is an *interpersonal* phenomenon and argued that the
therapist should not interpret it in an all-or-nothing fashion: "The
feelings that patients struggle with are highly charged, painful,
conflict-laden areas of human experience for the therapist as well as
the patient" (p. 30). The crucial difference is not that the competent
therapist does not have fears and conflicts (Masterson's fallacy) but
that "because of greater psychological integration resulting from his
own developmental experiences and analysis, [he] is less frightened
of, and less prone to run from, these feelings than is the patient" (p.
31). Other, still less obvious ways in which I used projective identification to escape the unit's pressures will emerge in my critique of
the concept.

Irrespective of the flaws in my definition, projective identification
played an important and constructive role in my psychotherapy with
Kay. Not only did it salvage my pride and help me to forgive myself
for my rebellious emotions, but it suggested a new conception of my
practice and a strategy for proceeding. The notions of containing,
tolerating, and digesting Kay's feelings were particularly suggestive.
In the next section of this chapter I illustrate and discuss how they
influenced what I did.

TOLERATING, CONTAINING, AND DIGESTING
FEELINGS

As my training year at State drew to a close, Kay and I took an
increasingly retrospective view of our relationship. I recorded in my

therapy notes one such reminiscent moment on Kay's part shortly following her belligerent announcement that soon I would be moving on "to bigger and better things":

> She is certain that I care about her because (1) she's helping me to get my [doctorate in psychology] and (2) because of the time she slammed a chair against the wall and I stuck with her even though she could tell I was frightened. All in all, [she says], I put up with her—all her bitching and yelling, etc. [from 6/18].

I vividly remembered Kay slamming the chair. I present it here as the most dramatic instance I can recall of my efforts to tolerate both her feelings and my own.[2]

Over the weekend of March 22 and 23, Kay, without consulting anyone, had pierced another set of holes in her ears (she already had three). Perhaps concerned that neither I nor the rest of the staff would respond to her behavior, she ostentatiously twirled her "diamond" studs throughout her Monday session with me and complained that her earlobes hurt a lot. I duly reported her possibly self-destructive—and certainly defiant—conduct to the head nurse; by our next session on Wednesday the latter had confiscated all of Kay's earrings. My notes on the session continue:

> She was furious and slammed a chair against the wall early in the session. Ranted and raved about how the staff's response was excessive. [Staff] should've taken only piercing earrings, not *all* of them. Hates State, etc. etc. Anger gave way gradually to sorrow/ self-pity. Earrings are her identity, what she's gotten for herself on her own. . . . At end of session apologized to me for slamming chair. Did not want me to think she was angry at *me*.

In this exchange my sense of vulnerability was indisputably my own: when Kay slammed the chair, I was afraid of being physically assaulted and hurt. By investigating the significance of her angry response, however, I think I can plausibly suggest that my fears echoed hers.

---

[2] While I tried to explore with Kay her apprehensions that I was abandoning her because she was not good enough, a more thoroughgoing Kleinian psychotherapist might have viewed her phrasing of the memory as a compliment and as her attempt to make reparations for her earlier hostile and envious attacks on the "good" (or "goods") that I represented.

The key to my interpretation came from Kay herself: because she equated her earrings (and, more generally, her physical appearance) with her "self," she held me responsible for what she experienced as an assault on her life. Her threat of bodily violence against me answered in kind her understanding of my attack upon her. More subtly, moreover, Kay was also fundamentally challenging my identity as a clinician. While perhaps not as essential to my self-definition as Kay's earrings were to hers, my clinical judgment was nonetheless central to my self-esteem. When Kay condemned the excessiveness of the staff's response (instigated by me), she was fundamentally challenging my rationale for my actions. This complemented her experience of my sabotaging of her "self."

As much as I still consider plausible these equivalences between my own and Kay's feelings, my newly articulated value on containing them checked my impulse to make them explicit to her. Nor did I call for assistance from the staff or cut short the session. Sufficiently assured that Kay had attacked a chair and not me (and that, beneath the storminess of the moment, we had enough of an alliance), I did nothing beyond staying with her. What ensued, in fact, justified the silent interpretation I had made. Seemingly reassured that we could manage our feelings, Kay quickly calmed down. With the safety supplied by my emotionally holding her together, by session's end she could accept and reflect on the fears that were her own. It seems possible, moreover, that her apology and protestation that she was not angry at *me* evidenced a recovery from the blurring of our emotions—and our boundaries—which had earlier been dominant.

With severely disturbed individuals, Ogden urges that it is best, more often than not, to accept quietly the powerful feelings they arouse. Given this basic therapeutic attitude, spoken interpretions to the patient are less important and may, in certain cases, indicate the therapist's acting out. In other words, even if one's formulation is right, voicing it before a patient can hear it may covertly communicate one's own hostility or fear that the patient is "too hot to handle."[3] As Ogden put it:

> Processing the projective identification without acting upon the engendered feelings is an essential aspect of the therapeutic process.

---

[3] Stephen Lerner (1979) made a similar argument, without specifically using the concept of projective identification, in an article entitled, "The Excessive Need to Treat."

> . . . Acceptance of the projected aspects of the patient as a communi-
> cation to be understood—as opposed to proddings or assaults to be
> acted upon or fled from—constitutes the background of the thera-
> peutic situation [p. 54].

When Kay frightened me by slamming the chair, projective identification provided me with a psychotherapeutic stance that enabled
me to stand firm despite my temptation to flee.

Up until this point in my training, I had assumed that interpretation was the definitive activity of a psychoanalytic psychotherapist.
The clinical phenomenon referred to as projective identification
now presented me with a new possibility and set of problems about
how best to proceed. As much as the concept freed me to tolerate
my own feelings, it unsettled my sense of what I was supposed to do.
It was one thing to assert that Kay had put her feelings into me, it was
quite another to contemplate what it meant to digest and then feed
them back. Was it possible that I might just sit back and do nothing
indefinitely? Wouldn't that surely be too passive and not nourishing
enough for Kay? Perhaps I might tell her how *I* felt in our interactions? The implied risk of impropriety was both dangerous and
tempting. Increasingly aware of the ambiguities of the psychotherapeutic relationship, I struggled to clarify what balance to strike.

Given these uncertainties, what I actually tried out ranged from
cautious and well-considered interpretations to off-the-cuff retorts. I
grew increasingly daring—or perhaps foolhardy—as time went on.
At the more conservative end of these new possibilities were observations I made to Kay of my role's "responsiveness" to hers, a
phenomenon I loosely affiliated with projective identification.[4] Let
me illustrate what I mean.

As the treatment progressed, I grew increasingly curious about
what it meant that Kay so frequently demanded that I tell her what to
talk about. Sometimes her question followed an exchange in which
she evidently felt wronged or misunderstood. At these times, she
seemed to use it to signify that she was ceasing her involvement in

---

[4] Joseph Sandler (1976) developed the notion of role responsiveness in an article
entitled, "Countertransference and Role Responsiveness." "Although not directly
addressing the entire set of phenomena encompassed by the concept of projective
identification," according to Ogden (1982), role responsiveness does make an
"important contribution to our thinking about the interpersonal effects of one's
unconscious psychological state" (p. 80).

our conversation. Most of the time, though, "So what should I talk about?" was her opening line, spoken with varying affect from sullen to coy. Given my own preoccupation with how I should conduct myself, I wondered if she, too, was seeking clues to her identity.

When I answered by telling Kay that we could discuss this or that expectation of the team's (for example, that she should look at why she so frequently squabbled with her peers), it seemed that she responded in one of two ways. Either she redoubled her condemnation of the system that oppressed her, or she strove to do whatever was necessary in order to be released. Contemplating these responses in light of our relationship, I decided that with them Kay was often casting me as the pimp whom she alternately resented or sought to please. When she experienced herself as coerced and victimized, she made me feel like her pimp-enslaver. When, alternately, she fancied herself seductive and desirable, she acted with me as if I were her pimp-protector.

As before, Kay herself planted the seed to my interpretation. In the winter months she complained bitterly of her prostitution and her hospitalization as if they were alike. I first made this analogy explicit in mid-January, and she readily agreed. Encouraged that I was on to something, I pursued it further, wondering specifically about its implications for our interactions. Working from my own feelings as well as from what Kay said, in subsequent sessions I began suggesting that she was reenacting with me her old patterns of behaving. On February 28, for example, in a session immediately following our second appearance before the judge, we began with a standoff that I interpreted as consistent with my line of reasoning:

Kay began by being quiet. Then asked what I wanted her to talk about. Silence. Asked again. Silence. Asked again. I commented on how that question presumed that she needed to figure out what *I* wanted, that she needed to give me *my* "pleasure." She was irritated, wanted "clear and direct answers." I said there was no clear and direct answer to that question [of what she should talk about] . . . [Berated me for giving the judge "a line of bullshit."] Shifted to how I let her down. I'd said to the judge that she'd made progress, but made it sound like she wasn't doing as much as she could. . . . [Complained about the slowness of discharge planning.] She said, how can we know when she'll be ready to leave if we don't have questions with clear and direct answers? I said, it's hard but something we'd work out together.

When Kay clamored for unambiguous answers and accused me of letting her down, I felt manipulated, as if I might really be as powerful (and yet as paradoxically impotent and constrained) as she would have me believe. This recognition—of a way of feeling that Kay evoked in me—then became the impetus for what I said to her. Wanting to free myself from the limitations that I felt she had thrust upon me, I made explicit that I did not have the answers that she so adamantly wanted. I rejected her disturbing attributions of my omnipotence and helplessness and hoped that in doing so I was simultaneously freeing up new possibilities for our being together.

In sum, my first clinical application of projective identification stopped just short of actually admitting to the countertransference that informed it. As time went on, instead, I loosened up, commenting in the sessions on how I was feeling in an effort to get at what was going on with Kay. This was most evident in a running debate that we had, throughout March and April, about whether or not I would allow her to read her chart. Unable to get a satisfactory idea of what the team thought of her in face-to-face conversations, she apparently presumed that the written records would hold the secrets she so desired. Without denying her request (as we both knew, she had a legal right to her record), I insisted that we examine what she was looking for and what it would mean to her to find it out.

After several sessions in which she angrily refused to tell me anything, I used my own experience of being shut out to initiate a change of tactics:

> I tried explaining my feelings to Kay about our interaction, beginning with how I couldn't understand what was going on with her unless she helped me out. She announced with grim satisfaction that that's how *she* feels; she wants me to feel what she feels, viz, rejected, hurt, confused. Intense experience, but genuine. Kay wanting to understand what people think of her, what she thinks of herself, and feeling she can't get help/can't do this [from March 21].

In this instance, directly revealing my experience had yielded apparently positive results: Kay was more willing to examine with me her motivations for and feelings about having access to her chart. My adaptation of projective identification seemed validated: emotions evoked in me had resonated with those of my patient. By making them explicit, we were more able than we had been to communicate directly about them.

In the following session, I did allow Kay to review her chart, an act that had more serious repercussions for me on the unit than it seemed to have for Kay herself. I will save for chapter 5 a full account of what happened. Suffice it to say now that it did not predispose me to be as generous about showing Kay her chart again.[5] In fact, for several weeks, we barely mentioned the issue. In all likelihood, my having been chastised was evident to her. On April 23, however, as I was walking through the unit's "day area," Kay shouted out that she wanted me to bring her chart to session. Embarrassed, I informed her that we had to discuss her request further. Impervious to my discomfort, she persisted until I left the room. Later she began our session with a resumption of her request. Mightily uncomfortable with what felt like pressure from all sides, I neither anticipated nor rehearsed the sharpness with which I replied to her insistence:

> Session began on the same demanding note and I responded with felt irritation; told Kay that I found it offensive to be treated like that [viz, ordered around on the unit] and that she should know by now that something as complicated as reading charts had to be talked about. After a few exchanges she gave up, saying, "Let's just drop it then!" Demanded to know what I wanted to talk about. Impasse. I then asked about her response to my getting angry. [She replied,] "I'm used to it. . . . At least now I know you're human!"

I do not think that this argument exemplifies my patient's projec-tive identification; if anything, it demonstrates how I displaced my own pique with the team onto her. The session as a whole, though, does reflect my growing tolerance for what I was feeling, which I consider an indirect benefit of what I had learned from projective identification generally. For better or worse, I could begin to ac-knowledge that my emotions played a central role in what we needed to work out. I did not conclude despairingly—as I would have earlier—that my unresolved conflicts spelled doom for my career. Nor did I run away from my discomfort by pretending that I could

---

[5] Ironically, my being scolded for acting without consulting the team coincided with Kay's being scolded for having pierced her ears. This demonstrates not only that therapists are not immune to acting out but that a notion of "parallel process" may provide a more parsimonious account of what happened.

blame my outburst totally on what Kay had evoked. Armed, instead, with a more positive conception of countertransference, I encouraged the two of us as best I could to look at the relationship that involved us both.

This relative loosening up of what I allowed myself to feel and to talk about in my interactions with Kay is more evident when compared with our angry sessions in the fall. As already described at length in chapter 2, Kay's running away from the hospital was a blow to my self-confidence that yielded unpleasant doubts and a keen sense of betrayal. Overlaying my response was my conviction that none of it was acceptable; a more seasoned and secure therapist, I believed, would remain unruffled and detached. Thus, even though I could not hide my temper from Kay in our sessions, I would not admit it openly. In fact, if confronted, I might well have denied it. From the perspective of projective identification, Kay was fully justified in accusing me of being withholding, in a particularly contentious session four days after her return. Because of my own repudiation then of what I was feeling, I excluded my own emotions from the collaborative consideration I later thought they deserved.

Ogden, attempting to clarify when an interpretation of projective identification seems justified, wrote the following:

> Not all mental activity or feeling states of the therapist reflect the internal state of the patient. In attempting to determine the presence or absence of interpersonal pressure describable in terms of projective identification, the therapist's immediate and retrospective sense that he has been limited in the range of feelings, ideas, and self-images available to him is central. Interventions based on inferences made from an analysis of the therapist's intrapsychic state [are] not validated by the succeeding events of the therapy session or of the following sessions [p. 148].

As these examples demonstrate, I defined projective identification even more loosely and applied it generously to a diverse range of interactions. It served an important purpose in my practicing, providing a place for my emotions within my relationship with Kay.

By recasting countertransference in a more positive light, projective identification helped me to "redesign" (as Schön might say) problems posed to me by my psychotherapeutic work. Using it to reflect on my interactions with Kay, I was newly able to make sense of what had before been uncertain. In place of Masterson's censure of unresolved conflicts, I put what Erikson (1964) called "disciplined subjectivity," "[the inclusion] in [the psychotherapist's] field of observation [of] a *specific self-awareness* in the very act of perceiving his patient's actions and reactions" (p. 54; italics Erikson's). This did not mean, however, that I rejected outright Masterson's theory of the borderline adolescent. At a time when gaining perspective on Kay's history and illness was of paramount importance, his characteriza-tion of who she was had been indispensable, and the narrative structure he provided continued, over the course of her treatment, to shape how I understood her.

What I challenged, instead, were Masterson's views on the thera-pist's expertise and objectivity. His implicit claim that the therapist has the right answers, coupled with his insistence that the therapist remain emotionally uninvolved, was contradicted by my experience at State. My psychotherapeutic role was far more ambiguous, open-ended, and bound up with my patient's than Masterson's perspective would ever allow. Instead of assuming, as he does, that clinical acumen becomes compromised by one's own subjectivity, I came to argue that the latter is a foundation on which therapeutic expertise builds. Projective identification provided me with a vocabulary and theoretical rationale that made this argument possible.

Constructively applied, projective identification brought my thinking closer to what I felt and did. But when used defensively, it generated its own set of difficulties. As much as it provided me with much-needed room to move, I also used it to idealize and perpetuate my relative isolation from the unit. Drawing on the metaphor of an unholy alliance, I will develop this critique in concluding the chapter.[6] I argue that what seemed at first to be so magically efficacious drew some of its potency from what it shielded me from.

UNHOLY ALLIANCES

My adaptation of a notion of projective identification provided immediate solutions to the problems that tormented me in the

---

[6] McCaughan (1985) used Keith's (1968) metaphor of "unholy alliance" to describe patterns of adaptation and defense typical of the novice adolescent psychotherapist. My own misalliance closely ressembled what he called a "flight into the therapy." What I want to stress here, though, is how I felt justified in isolating myself because of the ideas I adopted.

weeks following Kay's running away from State. Most important, it reversed my self-condemnation and significantly tempered my wish to give up. With a renewed sense of confidence about what I could accomplish, I felt more positive about my training and committed to carrying it through.

My improved relationship with Kay, though, came at a cost. An overly exclusive focus on projective identification allowed me to feel superior to and apart from the staff on the unit and my State supervisor in ways that compromised the psychotherapeutic goals that I had set out to accomplish. For all intents and purposes, I stubbornly resisted coordinating my efforts with theirs. Spinning a cocoon around "my" patient and ideas, I presumed to rise above the poor relationships that I had with them. As subsequent experience made all too evident, I was self-deluded in thinking that I could be successful without their support.

My romanticized embrace of an outsider status had at least three aspects that I can now identify. First of all, I was indulging a fascination with Melanie Klein, herself an outsider to American psychiatry, whose provocative language, coupled with the passionate condemnation she aroused, seemed to give voice and meaning to my unhappy experience. Second, I used this special and esoteric identification to affiliate myself with those earlier supervisors from whom I had learned of projective identification while discounting what I might gain from in-house clinicians. Finally, by concentrating so intently on what Kay "put into" me and how to "digest" it, I could pay lip service to my State supervisor's request that I "turn down the noise," even as I quietly clung to my conviction that he could not appreciate complexity. In the following pages I will look more closely at these facets of my unholy alliance, showing how they converged in my avoidance of the context in which Kay and I worked.[7]

---

[7] As Nancy Kulish (1985-1986) pointed out in her comprehensive review article, projective identification is also vulnerable to a number of other critiques. Among those she discussed were the following points: (1) over the years the concept, so variously defined, has become overburdened; (2) a therapist may use it to rationalize countertransference "as being evoked by his patient" (p. 98); (3) the concept has become "concretized, so that writers speak as if . . . thoughts leap about mysteriously in the air from one psyche to another" (p. 100); and (4) projective identification all too often confounds competing models of the mind and thus leads to "irreconcilable visions of the human condition" (p. 102). In contrast to Kulish's survey, my own critique follows more closely the logic of my own "reflection-in-action."

I saw my position on the unit as homologous, in some respects, to what I understood of Melanie Klein's in this country. In my educational experience, her theories of child development and psychoanalysis had attracted only grudging recognition for their importance in the history of psychotherapy; far more frequently, critics greeted them skeptically, if not with open hostility.[8] Given my own sense of being unappreciated at State, I felt a sympathetic, if distant, alliance with this theorist who was similarly undervalued.

What appealed to me most, though, about Klein and her followers was the language that they used in their formulations. Their talk was unabashedly raw and visceral; it seemed somehow more suited than other psychological dialects to the unadulterated stuff of the unconscious. *Digesting* and *horrible bloody mish-mash*—to say nothing of *attacking, biting, tearing,* and any number of broken body parts—the words themselves were evocative of what I imagined Kay's experience to be.

Kay had a particular preoccupation with her body's integrity that the Kleinian idiom aptly captured. Alongside her insistence that she was beautiful and desirable were never-ending fears that inside she was ugly or rotten. Her chart documents how frequently she had the doctor called to deal with her aches and pains; our sessions made her worries more vivid. She had a preoccupation with pregnancy; possibly she fantasized that babies could fill up the emptiness inside her. At other times, she was afraid that a penis could attack and harm her. Menstrual blood not only confirmed that she had lost the fantasized baby but also was proof that some part of her was "broken."

Kay also fantasized herself as dangerous and destructive in her relationships with others. A dream she had toward the end of our work combined a number of her concerns. She described the dream after telling me what she would miss about me and after stating that she would refuse a new therapist. According to my therapy notes:

---

[8] Although I did not know it at the time, even Ogden (1982), an apologist for an essentially Kleinian idea, betrayed antipathy when discussing the theorist herself. He obviously acknowledged that projective identification owes its genesis and development to Klein and her followers, citing Bion, in particular, as relevant to his formulation of the concept. When discussing Klein herself his tone shifted remarkably. He stated that, its origins notwithstanding, "projective identification has *no* inherent connection with *any* aspect of specifically Kleinian metapsychology or clinical theory" (p. 76, italics added). My aim here is not to argue for or against Ogden's claim per se but, rather, to illustrate the vehemence with which even the most evenhanded of critics can reject Klein's views.

Had nightmares last night (now *really* manic). In the first, the pimple on her face was real swollen, so she went to the doctor who lanced it and a *bug* crawled out—and all this pus. The doctor cut the bug in half—a "pusbug"—it was *gross!*

The dream admits of several interpretations within the context of our relationship. At the time, I thought Kay was acknowledging her inner ugliness, which I, the doctor, had uncovered. Equally plausibly, she could have been attributing the ugliness to an alien other that had invaded her life and that she wanted to expel. What intrigued me was the dream's primitive imagery of the messiness of inside and out. My own struggle to make sense of projective identification seemed illuminated by such images, themselves enhanced by a Kleinian language.

I continue to value how a Kleinian vocabulary has enriched my psychological understanding. Problems arose, though, to the extent that I mastered the idiom to set myself apart from those with whom I worked. I assumed that I knew a better, secret language that gave me access to truths about my patient that the staff could not imagine. By using projective identification to justify my retreat from my supervisor and the team, I established an unholy alliance with Kay that ultimately could not stand.

In what McCaughan (1985) characterized as a "flight into the therapy," I withdrew my concern from the team I was part of and concentrated on deciphering Kay's unconscious communications. Even this would not have been so detrimental if I had made some effort to communicate to others what I had learned. Instead, under the guise of doing my job as Kay's psychotherapist, I disparaged the indispensability of teamwork within the hospital setting.

I fantasized that I had become initiated into an exclusive and select society composed of three favored former supervisors. Whereas no one at State, it seemed, was concerned about my misery, these absent others had generously provided me with the fresh perspective I needed. Significantly, one of these supervisors, an intense, very dynamic woman, had completed analytic training at the Tavistock Clinic in London and felt sensitive to her own outsider status in the States. Another, my adviser, attracted me with his independence of mind, his thoughtful refusal to adopt any one "party line." Thus, when my former supervisors described the paradoxical phenomenon of projective identification, I was not only enthralled by its strangeness and intensity but eager to engage in conversations about it with such fascinating people. My actual experience of projective identification in working with Kay, as I have attempted to demonstrate in this chapter, confirmed the concept's value. I renewed my gratitude to these talented supervisors, though, by smugly scorning my State supervisor's lack of sophistication.

As I have already discussed in chapter 2, I had a decidedly uneasy alliance with my State supervisor, whom I experienced as incapable of tolerating and containing my anxieties about training. I felt personally rebuffed and misunderstood when he told me that he wanted me to talk less about the unit and more about Kay in her sessions, and so my anger at the unit staff extended to him. At best, I feared that my intensity overwhelmed this man, despite his years of experience as a clinician and clinical administrator at State; at worst, I devalued him as unempathic and rigid.

When my supervisor complained that there was too much "noise" during our supervisory sessions that fall, I took this criticism much to heart, as if here again I was guilty of not remaining calm, cool, and collected, traits that, according to Masterson, were required to avoid the pitfalls of countertransference. Projective identification gave me a way of defending myself against this perceived censure. Yes, there *was* noise, I granted him that, but it was not the sort of static that he implied. Instead, it was the "bloody mish-mash" of Kay's unconscious and thus essential to the treatment. If my supervisor only knew how to deal with this complexity, I thought, then he would stop nagging me to "turn it down." By shifting my ideal from unruffled and knowing assertiveness to a degree of comfort with blurred boundaries, I effectively—if covertly—repudiated him. Under the guise of complying with his instruction to talk more exclusively about Kay's psychotherapy, I withdrew my attention and respect, at least for a time.

Over time, I have not decided that my State supervisor's notion of psychotherapy was right nor that what my former supervisors taught me was wrong. For all that I legitimately emulated in my previous teachers, though, I think that in this instance my loyalty was misguided and unfortunate. I aligned myself with them—all outside of the hospital—and used this fantasized alliance to rationalize the separateness I felt inside the hospital. My identification with idealized and absent others, in other words, covertly contributed to my isolation from my hospital colleagues, whom, I reassured myself, I did not need because I had something much better. Because I almost never talked to my supervisor or teammates about my special knowledge, I preserved the cocoon that my secret allegiance pro-vided me.

I did not talk, but my actions did, and it was to these that the milieu "talked back." Without consulting the team, I made impor-tant decisions about Kay's treatment, such as showing her her chart. Immediately confronted, I found that my fragile defense—that I was better than all of them—crumbled when they scolded me. Similarly, the responsiveness of the nurses and psychiatric aides rudely proved false the illusion that Kay and I could do our work without them. For a time, I tried to recover my unholy alliance, but eventually it proved too vulnerable. I needed a better way to make sense of the unit and of my place within it.

Like Masterson's theory of the borderline adolescent, projective identification is neither all-right nor all-wrong. At its best, it is a point of view on a set of complicated interactions. As such, it genuinely furthered my work with Kay, providing me with new interpretative possibilities, enhanced self-esteem, and greater room within which to move. My alliance with the idea became unholy, though, when I used it to justify an overly limited conception of psychotherapy. I kept the staff's and my supervisor's opinions too far at bay and pretended a superior knowledge. Most seriously, I denied how much both Kay and I depended on the unit's structure and stability.

In the next chapter I describe how I came to see this depen-dence—or interdependence—as an asset. Drawing on a wide-ranging literature about the multidirectional network of hospital treatment, I could redefine my role as a therapist in a way that constructively included my relationships to the team. In so doing, to return to Schön's (1983) idiom, I was able to arrive "at a deeper and broader coherence of artifact and idea" (p. 164).

5

SHARED WORDS

While psychiatric hospitals generally realize that patients'
needs demand cohesion of the institution, even very good
hospitals fail to recognize that, to function best in their
own and the patient's interests, the staff needs the
institution's cohesiveness every bit as much as the
patients.
Bruno Bettelheim, *A Home for the Heart*

My difficulties practicing psychotherapy within a hospital milieu began almost as soon as I arrived for my training at State. Within a week the unit had assigned me two patients (who had already been hospitalized for several months) and a treatment team (Team B) with which I was to coordinate their care. At my first team meeting, others warned me that one of my patients, a 16-year-old girl diagnosed as a "borderline with depressive features," was a "splitter." In the following few days this caution, repeated frequently by various milieu staff and especially by the young psychiatrist who was my team's leader, heightened my sense of danger and bewilderment; the adolescent herself seemed harmlessly sad, and I had little idea what I was supposed to be guarding against.

After about two weeks of confused apprehension, I approached the nurse supervisor, a regular member of my team, and hesitantly confessed that when the team leader warned of my patient's "splitting," I did not understand what she meant. She greeted my admission with an unsmiling gaze and the dire pronouncement that it was not my patient but *I* who was guilty of "splitting." Stunned, I burst into tears and then began blubbering about how new everything was to me and how vulnerable I felt. In contrast to her censure of my first complaint, the nurse supervisor responded kindly to my crying, handing me a box of Kleenex and offering to make me coffee. I left her office vaguely comforted but still in the dark. If anything, I felt that I had become split off from the team of which I was a part.

The confusion, shame, and, eventually anger that characterized this initial encounter with my colleagues formed what I have called the "noisy" backdrop to my early months at State. Harold Searles (1979), in a chapter entitled "Paranoid process among members of the therapeutic team," captured my experience when he wrote that the inpatient psychotherapist commonly fears "that this whole unembraceably vast vortex was less a team, or even a collection, of separate human individuals than a giant unicellular organism which threatened to engulf any individual who came into contact with it" (p. 90). My introduction to the milieu literature, half a year later, marked a turning away from this paranoid position.

Improved relationships with staff and supervisor alike were the unexpected but welcome benefit of the reading course, directed by my graduate school adviser, that I began when I was on Christmas vacation far away from the hospital. I read a book aptly titled *The End of Hope* (Kobler and Stotland, 1964); this story of a rash of suicides on an inpatient psychiatric ward, seemingly linked to the *staff's* sense of hopelessness, made me curious about the interpersonal dynamics of the staff on A-2. In subsequent weeks I pursued this new interest, surveying the variety of works written about the psychiatric hospital as an institution, as a training facility, and as a therapeutic modality. A growing appreciation for the fact that my work took place in a context or milieu gradually tempered my own hopelessness in the face of the unit's "interference." My newfound perspective on the diversity of interactions and purposes that constitute a hospital unit made me more tolerant of my colleagues and contributed to an easing of the tensions between us.

Reading next Stanton and Schwartz's (1954) classic, *The Mental Hospital*, together with related books and articles, helped my practicing primarily by making explicit how individual psychotherapists within a hospital must guage and coordinate their efforts within the realistic constraints and possibilities of the context and relationships in which they operate. Perhaps ironically, the milieu literature also reintroduced me to the interpersonalist perspective that had originally attracted me to psychoanalytic psychotherapy. Stanton and Schwartz, a psychiatrist and sociologist, respectively, had both studied with Harry Stack Sullivan and conducted their research at The Chestnut Lodge, which Sullivan had directed for several years. Rather than limit their focus to the ways in which a patient's difficulties reveal themselves in the relationship to a therapist, however, Stanton and Schwartz broadened their framework to include more multifaceted systems.

Once I had encountered the possibility that such things as financial management, community relations, and staff morale could significantly affect a patient's psychiatric symptoms, the physical and interpersonal configuration of my workplace gained prominence in my thinking. I appraised my surroundings with new eyes, scrutinizing what I had barely noticed before. This chapter begins with a similar review—of the hospital unit, its organization, personnel, and patients.[1] Following this, I discuss more precisely what I found especially helpful about the milieu literature that I read. Drawing particularly on the concepts of the split social field and parallel process, I examine the practical consequences of this more comprehensive viewpoint, both for understanding Kay's difficulties on the unit and for understanding my own. While more inclusive in important respects than the viewpoints offered by theories either of the borderline or of projective identification, a milieu perspective was no more the right way to conceptualize the case than they were. In concluding the chapter I analyze A-2's ritualized good-byes to patients and therapists who were leaving as an example of how the increasing cohesion that rewarded my new perspective also curtailed my advocacy for what Kay needed psychotherapeutically.

WHERE I WAS, WHO I WAS WITH

State Hospital is an oddly shaped, 11-story brick building located amidst a poorly conceived conglomeration of highways, hospitals,

---

[1] A much fuller description of a similar unit and its treatment philosophy can be found in Marohn, Dalle-Molle, McCarter, and Linn's (1980) *Juvenile Delinquents: Psychodynamic Assessment and Hospital Treatment.*

and low-income housing in a large Midwestern city. Neither ugly nor elegant, it was built solely to serve a purpose: the care of those mentally disturbed individuals who could not afford to go elsewhere. In earlier years it had renown also as a research institution, but funding cuts had sharply limited these activities by 1985, when I arrived there. It continued, however, to be an important training site for mental health professionals, with medical residents and psychology and social work students regularly spending from six months to a year there.

A-2 was one of three adolescent units in the hospital; all the others served adults. Like the hospital itself, the unit was far more functional than attractive, with uncarpeted linoleum floors and painted cement-block walls. A glassed-in nurses' station had full view of the hallway, off which were 15 single bedrooms, 2 washrooms, a small kitchen, an examination room, and the activities therapists' office. The nurses could also watch, off to one side, the large common room or "day area." Out of view, down a shorter hallway, were the music room (which also served as a meeting room for family conferences and my team, Team B), the activities shop, and the head nurse and nurse supervisor's offices. The unit chief's office was on the same floor, but at a distance from the unit, while the assistant unit chief's office (seldom used) was on another floor altogether.

The physical space, crowded with patients and staff, fostered an abiding atmosphere of too much to do with not enough resources. The chatter and clutter of the nurses' station, in many ways the hub of the unit, was bewildering to a newcomer. Everyone seemed to be complaining or joking, often at the expense of the patients. For weeks I had only the vaguest notion of what I overheard discussed in deceptively familiar, but idiosyncratically used terms, such as *working*, *inappropriate behavior*, *limits*, *set ups*, *acting out*, and the ubiquitous *splitting*. Other terms—such as *FLRs*, *PALs*, and *TPRs*[2]—were altogether mystifying. Between the staff's apparent cynicism and the secret language they shared, I and the other trainees felt that our welcome was perfunctory. Only later could I try to reconstruct what our arrival meant to the permanently employed nurses and mental health workers (or "milieu staff").

Not only did the A-2 nursing and milieu staff work very hard but

---

[2] Full leather restraints, passalongs, and treatment progress reviews respectively.

they organized their collective identity around being tough and competent. To their way of thinking, they were underpaid and overtaxed but *damn* good. During the summer I arrived, they had quelled a near-riot on the unit upstairs, and they were responsible for retraining yet another unit's staff. In general, their referring to themselves as a unified staff—as opposed to separate groups of nurses and psychiatric assistants—emphasized their sense of cohesiveness and conviction about their importance to the patients' treatment.[3]

Representatives from the nursing and milieu staff played an important role on the two treatment teams (Team A and Team B) that also included a psychiatrist (as team leader), a social worker, a recreational therapist, and a number of individual therapists. While I doubt that any had had much formal training in milieu therapy, under the strong leadership of the nurse supervisor the unit employees did define their work in terms of therapeutic aims that depended on close coordination with other team members. Briefly put, the staff understood that a patient's treatment occurred not only in psychotherapy sessions but in his or her relationship to the unit-based community or milieu as well. Thus, from the staff's point-of-view, patients were helped just as much (if differently) by talking about infractions of rules or the feasibility of new privileges as they were by exploring the more dynamic reasons for how they felt and behaved. Indeed, not only were the staff convinced that they could manage patients that no other hospital could, but they smugly maintained that they knew a lot more than the trainees who came and went. For all the truth to these claims, though, the staff's pride and stoicism overlay more complicated emotions.

To all intents and purposes, the nurses and milieu staff were the ones who stayed behind. Having been left by innumerable trainees, patients, and administrators over the years, they were keenly sensitive to being seduced and abandoned. The unit chief in 1985 was young, new, and scarcely out of training himself. He had become

---

[3] From my perspective as a trainee the nurses and milieu workers constituted a cohesive group or staff despite my awareness that nurses had a higher status and greater authority in the hospital hierarchy. I suspect now that each subgroup had a stronger sense of identity as a nurse or milieu worker respectively and that there may have been interstaff rivalries. However, I continue to believe that these subgroups shared a strong and fundamental sense of common purpose that justified my frequently referring to them as a single staff.

unit chief very abruptly the previous February when his predecessor, a senior clinician, had accepted a more prestigious position and given 24 hours notice. Already relatively uncertain and inexperienced, the new chief's overnight promotion made him an easy target for the staff's justified anger at the leader who had abandoned them. Unfortunately, they blamed their current administrator for anything from too much paperwork to patient violence.[4] The assistant unit chief was more assertive, organized, and seasoned, but because she worked only 20 hours a week, staff perceived her, too, as generally ineffective. Thus, both the unit chief and the assistant unit chief, the titular heads of the unit's two treatment teams, frequently failed to hold the staff's respect and attention. Very quickly, I decided that the nurse supervisor was in charge, but this was not a topic that anyone would openly discuss.

Although the unit was supposed to have no more than 15 patients at a time, the threat of going "over census" was ever present. In fact, during my 12 months there, this happened rarely; still, the staff feared the worst and painted dreadful pictures of therapy rooms and offices being used for the overflow. As part of a state institution with a defined catchment area, the unit was obliged to admit any adolescent who met certain criteria. Much of the chief social worker's job was deflecting admissions and finding alternative placements. Whenever the unit actually admitted a patient, the staff's griping escalated, as if this new admission might finally be the back-breaking straw.

Unquestionably, the patients were very difficult and demanding. Most were impulsive and delinquent, and not a few could be violent; almost all had undergone hospitalization at least once before. Kay's childhood was not unique for its abuse and instability; most of the adolescents had been brutalized in one way or another. A few adolescents responded to their maltreatment predominantly with depression or psychosis, but for many more, overt rage was their most usual affect.

The unit staff's responsibility, as they saw it, was to keep a lid on misbehaviors and to stay in control. They always kept the unit locked and accompanied patients whenever they left (most often for

---

[4] Combining object relations theory with an appreciation of group processes and open systems, Otto Kernberg (1978b) argued persuasively that administrative organization on a psychiatric unit cannot simply be the fault of the unit leader's personality.

school, in the same building, two stories down). They gave "restrictions" liberally—for anything from sleeping late, to swearing, to threatening another person—and recorded them on a large board in the nurses' station, which everyone could see. The day-to-day consequences of these restrictions were, in fact, minimal. Because everyone generally regarded them as significant to a patient's overall progress, though, much of the staff's time with patients was organized around their "working off" these restrictions.

The place of individual psychotherapy on the unit was indeterminate at best. Even though the unit's purported philosophy made psychotherapy central to its work, several circumstances mitigated against a full implementation of these principles. At the most mundane level was the chronic problem of a shortage of therapy rooms, with complicated sign-up procedures for the one official room and the two nurses' offices frequently being proposed and revised throughout the year. Limited space complemented equally limited time. Therapists had to compete with school, occupational and recreational therapy, family therapy, quiet times, and study hours when scheduling each of their patient's thrice-weekly sessions, which were routinely limited to half an hour.

More fundamental than these actual constraints on conducting individual psychotherapy was the fact that all individual psychotherapists on A-2 were in training and thus part of the unit for at most a year. While it had not always been the case, at least for the year before my arrival, none of the permanent staff from psychiatry, social work, nursing, or the milieu worked as an individual therapist for any patient on the unit. Our not having private offices in which to work underscored the trainees' "transience." It was easy for the novice to feel inessential when confronted by such apparently palpable signs that State underrated psychotherapy.

There were, of course, many ways in which the unit encouraged us to get involved, but for a long time I was skeptical of the sincerity of these offers. Team meetings were an apt case in point. Although the team leaders told us psychotherapists-in-training that we were in charge of our patients' treatment, it soon became apparent that they subjected our direction to innumerable qualifications. For starters, the team discussed each patient for only 20 minutes a week, and issues of management—privileges, doctors' appointments, behavioral problems, and so forth—dominated much of this time. With no more than three or four minutes to discuss psychodynamics and treatment, I felt that the implicit message was that my efforts were less important.

In addition to attending team meetings and writing the requisite notes in our patients' charts, A-2 expected trainees to participate in morning and, preferably, afternoon "reports" on the patients from the milieu staff, weekly staff meetings and case conferences, and at least one milieu (or community) meeting with the patients each week. Staff repeatedly stressed the importance of leaving written notes, or "passalongs" for them in the nurses' station. Given our diffidence about how little we mattered, the overall participation of the psychotherapists was unenthusiastic and sporadic.

An especially difficult patient like Kay only exacerbated the uneasiness between the "transients" and the permanent staff. With these cases, conflicts over who knew best and who should be in charge intensified (although arguments were rarely direct and out in the open). While the psychotherapists were convinced that they best understood psychopathology, the staff grimly replied that they were the ones actually with the patients 24 hours a day.

My adoption of a more systemic way of interpreting these dis-agreements alleviated my tendency to take them personally, but it took some time before I fully realized its advantages. Indeed, I at first retreated to reading about other hospital settings in an effort to view my situation from afar. Applying my new understanding largely retrospectively, I reconstructed Kay's early hospitalization and treat-ment from the perspective of the milieu. My hypotheses were speculative, at times even fanciful, yet they introduced a flexibility to my thinking sorely lacking before. Gradually persuading myself that the unit was not an "unembraceably vast vortex," I was able to behave more generously on the job with my coworkers. In the following section, I will reflect more extensively on how this "rap-prochement" came about.

EMBRACING THE VAST VORTEX

I was introduced to the concept of a "split social field" by Stanton and Schwartz's *The Mental Hospital* (1954). Subtitled "A Study of Institutional Participation in Psychiatric Illness and Treatment," the book developed and defended the thesis that "the immediate envi-ronment is an important influence in the course of a patient's illness" (p. 6). The authors conducted a three-year sociopsychiatric study of the disturbed ward at Chestnut Lodge, an exclusive, long-term psychiatric facility, and concluded that unacknowledged discrepancies between formal and informal (or overt and covert) organizational purposes and procedures often result in an exacerbation of patient pathology. While not belittling the importance of a patient's relationship to the psychotherapist, their focus was on how administrative structure and the inpatient milieu effect change.

Given the intrastaff conflicts that had been focused on Kay, I became especially intrigued by a chapter in *The Mental Hospital* entitled, "Pathological Excitement and Hidden Staff Disagreement." The chapter carefully established in case after case how one could trace a severe deterioration in a patient's behavior to inconsistencies in treatment that had become systemic. In what they call a "mirror-image disagreement," the authors described how

> The two antagonists gradually narrowed their field of vision regarding the patient to one or a few general principles which they *agreed* to be the most important to the patient's management at the moment, but about which they held precisely opposite opinions. . . . The most frequent examples were: the patient should not be treated as a special case versus each patient should be treated according to his particular needs; the patient needs to be indulged a bit versus the patient needs to face "reality" and have less soft "unrealistic babying;" the symptom is "put on" and "can be stopped" versus the patient "cannot help it if he is sick;" the patient has "improved considerably" versus the patient is much "sicker" than he appears to be; the patient's hostility is "justified" versus it is "completely unjustified" [p. 359].

Reading this list of opposite opinions, I experienced a shock of recognition. While stereotypic and stripped down, many of these debates echoed those occasioned by Kay.

Even more interestingly, Stanton and Schwartz claimed that the controversial patient's extreme agitation frequently accompanied his "dissociation" or "splitting" of the staff who were feuding about him, a notion to which reading Masterson's theory of the borderline adolescent had already exposed me. Much like the patients described by Masterson, who divided the world into "all-good" and "all-bad," the pathologically excited patients at Chestnut Lodge perceived one caretaker as "friendly" and the other as "dangerous." For Stanton and Schwartz, however, the origin of this phenomenon is the opposite of what was proposed by Masterson. While the latter argued that splitting results from the patient's inability to coherently represent complex relationships, Stanton and Schwartz contended that the patient is responding to the "split social field":[5]

> The patient's dissociation was partially understandable in terms of the social situation which he faced. The two most immediately important persons in his life were, so to speak, pulling him in opposite directions, and each showed, while he continued doing this, that he, himself, was of a "divided mind" . . . If our hypothesis is correct that the patient's dissociation is a reflection of, and mode of participation in, a social field which is itself seriously split, it accounts for the sudden cessation of excitement following any resolution of this split in the social field [pp. 362-363].

By responding to his caretakers' conflicts with increasingly confused thinking and acting, the patient acts out or makes manifest the hidden discord between them. Once the staff discovers and makes explicit their disagreement, however, the patient's disturbed symptoms and splitting subsided rapidly.

Stanton and Schwartz's analysis complemented the case study of Crest Hospital by Kobler and Stotland (1964) in *The End of Hope*. From being a tightly organized institution with a strong emphasis on milieu therapy, this hospital became so embroiled in local politics that its administrative and financial security became—ultimately fatally—compromised. The staff, which had enjoyed a high level of self-confidence and self-esteem, gradually became demoralized in the face of the hospital's increasing dissolution. A vicious cycle ensued: patients responded to the staff's discouragement with exacerbated symptoms, which further plunged their caretakers into a conviction of their helplessness. Like Stanton and Schwartz, Kobler and Stotland contended that the staff covertly communicated their hopelessness to their wards, who then acted it out.

In a six-month period, five patients at Crest Hospital committed suicide. A sixth, who made an unsuccessful attempt and then

---

[5] The staff used the term "splitting" much more loosely than either Masterson or Stanton and Schwartz. For them, splitting referred most commonly to a patient's playing one staff member off against another but with the added assumption that the patient's capacity to generate interstaff conflict had everything to do with the patient's psychopathology and nothing to do with already existing disagreements or tensions among the staff.

transferred, later agreed to an interview with the authors. According to his own and the staff's recollections, in addition to extensive written documents, Joseph Ullman was depressed and anxious but by no means suicidal when first admitted to the hospital. Nonetheless, the staff soon became convinced of his suicidal potential and subjected him to numerous, yet inconsistent, suicidal "precautions." Over time, Mr. Ullman became persuaded that the staff *wanted* him dead and that they designed their insistence on his self-destructiveness, coupled with their lapses in watching him, to show him when and how to take his own life.

Together, the illustrations of the split social field phenomenon in *The End of Hope* and *The Mental Hospital* initiated a revolution in my thinking about working on A-2. The margins of my books are busy with enthusiastic comments and exclamation marks, and in longer course notes I began to speculate on how I was formulating Kay's case. In early February, for example, in my course notes I debated about the relative merits of two possible explanations for her running away three months before:

> [Either] Kay ran because she is a delinquent who cannot tolerate her own feelings [or] Kay ran because she perceived at some level that she was the center of conflict over whether or not she should stay and, when given opportunity, even invited, to run, did so as a "resolution" of interpersonal strife. . . . Need a perspective where both these views can be acknowledged.

As I continued to mull over the second hypothesis, the splits in the unit's social field seemed to proliferate.

Stanton and Schwartz (1954) did not argue that all disagreements are bad; indeed, to advocate such unanimity would likely breed covert dissension. Their focus, instead, was on conflicting viewpoints not acknowledged or even recognized; it is these hidden and undiscussed agendas that result in a patient's acting out. As they dryly observed, "The whole process in its middle stages [is] very, very quiet" (p. 344). Let me mention a few of the quiet controversies I came to suspect had a bearing on Kay.

My own disagreements with the team, I decided, were just the tip of the iceberg. Equally serious, and perhaps even more hidden, were conflicts between the milieu staff and the unit chief, between my team leader and the Children's Aid Society (CAS), and among members of the milieu staff. Since none of these were ever discussed openly in any detail, what follows can only be a series of educated guesses.

During my year at State, the milieu staff were perpetually angry at A-2's young unit chief. Kay arrived in the midst of an especially unhappy time. Not only had the former unit chief left precipitously in February 1985, but he had accepted a position that had oversight over several mental health institutions, including State Hospital. He (I learned very late in my year there) was directly responsible for A-2's staff being selected in the summer of 1985 to retrain another unit's staff in patient "external control" or behavioral management, a time-consuming task made all the more onerous because the staff justifiably feared that their peers, whose work had been found lacking by A-2's former boss, would resent them. Although, of course, they complied with what he demanded, the staff sullenly held the new unit chief responsible for not standing up to his predecessor.

The unit chief, feeling guilty, made a promise he could not keep: during the seven-week retraining period, the unit's census would not exceed 13. The staff, knowing full well that he did not have this authority, held him unrelentingly to his word in spite of its evident unfeasibility. The problem was not just that he admitted Kay in the midst of this sparring as the unit's 14th patient, but she was not even from the catchment area—she had had special connections. It would have been one thing, perhaps, if she had come from the neighborhood. Promises or no, the legal responsibility then would have been indisputable. But he had imported this obnoxious youth from a residential placement in *Maryland*! While no one ever voiced this resentment to me in so many words, it surely added to Kay's baggage and contributed to her not being liked.

The political strings that had been pulled chafed at my team leader as well, although not particularly because she had sympathy for the staff. During the first week that Kay was on A-2, I heard from a social worker that she might soon transfer to a longer-term adolescent unit, A-1, especially geared for juvenile delinquents who were wards of the state. I, of course, was angered by the possibility of losing so quickly my newest patient. I now think that the team leader was furious because she suspected that CAS was using her. For admission to A-1, an adolescent had to meet several criteria: he or she needed involvement with CAS and with the legal system and had to be already hospitalized. Application for Kay to this unit, in other words, could not have occurred from her placement in Maryland. Given the speed with which CAS initiated these proceedings once Kay was on A-2, it seems plausible that they saw her admission there as a stepping stone to the more specialized unit. In any event, when I complained to the team leader that *I* did not want Kay transferred, she curtly informed me, with no explanation, that the team would not be providing any documentation to CAS for their application to A-1. A woman who valued her own authority, she was letting me know that she, unlike the unit chief, was not someone whom people could push around.

Beneath these major, if unarticulated, tensions were other strains that contributed to the antipathy of each faction toward the recently arrived patient. The staff's already exceptional difficulties were compounded when they repeatedly had to assist the third, and newest, adolescent unit throughout the summer and fall of 1985. A-3's patients were especially violent, and, according to A-2's staff, their unit was especially ill-equipped to contain them. At one point a fire set on A-3 necessitated an evacuation of the entire hospital; at another, staff narrowly averted a patient riot. In both of these and several other less dramatic incidents, A-2's staff were instrumental in reining in the acting out. This additional work, coupled with the demanding patients already on A-2, practically guaranteed that they would not welcome a troublemaker like Kay.

The team leader's additional concerns had to do more specifically with the legal system. Kay had already sued CAS for their participation in the sex club; there was no guarantee that she would not someday sue State Hospital also. At that very moment, the team had become embroiled in a nasty legal fight with another patient's parents, who had threatened to bring a malpractice suit against the team leader. Understandably nervous, the last thing the team leader wanted was a second litigious case.

Further complicating this already complex web of attitudes and interactions was the dissension among the nursing and milieu staff about whether or not Kay was treatable. In part because of my own vulnerability as a newcomer and a novice, I failed to appreciate at the time the diversity of their opinions. Later in the year, however, when we were able to talk more freely, a milieu staff member confessed that he had never "pushed back on" (i.e., challenged) Kay because he did not want to waste his efforts on a "sociopath";

another member, who ended up working very closely with Kay, admitted that she felt particularly challenged by work with "borderlines." Even if they had shared their disagreements with me openly from the start, I do not think I would have heard them; I had yet to recognize the importance of the milieu. As it was, the staff refrained from challenging my assumption of their unanimity because of their own need to present themselves to the neophytes as a united front.

Uncovering the controversies that had quietly surrounded Kay's admission (and assuming, not unreasonably, that there were others that still eluded me), I considered the possibility that Kay had run away in response to *our* conflicts. Drawing on a concept of a split social field, I questioned how I had framed my earlier explanations solely in terms of a borderline adolescent's inability to contain her own mixed emotions and the intrastaff disagreements engendered by her projective identifications.[6] It seemed increasingly plausible, instead, that the controversies that surrounded her hospitalization were the source and not the result of her agitation and flight. Our dissension had less to do with her intrapsychic instability, in other words, than with the instabilities inherent in the interpersonal situation in which we placed her.

While my role in the hidden arguments was not so difficult to uncover, the concept of parallel process helped me to differentiate further my participation in the State Hospital system. Although various authors disagree about the mechanisms and extent to which it occurs, each of them use parallel process to identify how the events within an individual psychotherapy can become elucidated by paying attention to other interactions that bear upon it. Not unlike Stanton and Schwartz's notion of a mirror-image disagreement, parallel process explicates certain triangular relationships.[7] Instead of focusing on two staff members who disagree over a

---

[6] In my notes I approached the possibility that my use of projective identification precluded a thorough examination of interpersonal and situational contributions to Kay's difficulties when I wrote that "in a sense, resorting to projective identification was a *solution* for me—a way of talking to the staff about Kay and what she stirs up without accusing them of not liking her, etc. I talked about a kind of relationship in a way which absolved them—and me—from examining our own contribution [to her behavior]."

[7] In fact, Stanton and Schwartz (1954) anticipated parallel process when they analyzed the mechanisms of the mirror-image disagreement in terms of a "triangular process" between junior psychiatrists, their superiors, and patients under their joint care (see p. 360).

patient with whom they both work, parallel process typically explicates how a supervisee's relationship with a supervisor mirrors or
reenacts the relationship that the supervisee has with the patient.

According to Sachs and Shapiro (1976), for example, supervisees'
verbal recounting of a session to their supervisor is accompanied by
a more or less unconscious demonstration of what actually occurred. In effect, by evoking in the supervisor what they themselves
felt with their patient, the supervisees are able to communicate what
they cannot yet put into words. If supervisors, in turn, pay attention
to their own empathic responses, they can "infer what was going on
in the therapy by noticing what the therapist [is doing to them]" (p.
404).

Sachs and Shapiro (1976) explained parallel process in terms of
the novice practitioner's identification with the patient:

> It appears that identification often occurs when the novice therapist
> feels vulnerable and subject to anxiety at the same time that similar
> anxiety is being experienced by his patient who has problems in his
> life with which he cannot effectively cope. Potentially, there is a wide
> area of overlapping vulnerabilities between patients and inexperi-
> enced therapists who are both beset by doubts about their own
> capabilities and are fearful of being unequal to the therapeutic task
> [p. 407].

Arguing that these explanations are necessary but not sufficient,
Gediman and Wolkenfeld (1980) contended that even highly experienced and skilled supervisors can feel the sorts of vulnerabilities
that Sachs and Shapiro describe. Because "both patient and analyst
share a need *for* help; both analyst and supervisor share a need *to*
help; and all three share a concern with self-esteem issues" (p. 254),
Gediman and Wolkenfeld concluded that it is not the therapist's
level of expertise that is definitive but, rather, the structural and
dynamic similarities of psychoanalytic therapy and supervision.
Parallel process, in their view, is "truly triadic: a complex *multidirectional* network, or system, and not simply a unidirectional process
with a set point of origin in the patient" (p. 236).

McCaughan (1985) and Grey and Fiscalini (1987) took the concept one step further, broadening it to include any number of
interpersonal interactions in addition to those between supervisor
and supervisee. According to Grey and Fiscalini:

> Parallel process is a chain reaction that may occur in any intercon-
> nected series of interpersonal situations that are structurally and
> dynamically similar in significant respects. It is not limited to the
> supervisory situation. Typically it involves intertwined concerns
> about authority and dependency, and the participants' need to
> conceal their attempted solutions to those concerns, leading to an
> interlocking series of parallel transference-countertransference inte-
> grations [p. 131].

Specifically addressing parallelisms within an adolescent inpatient
setting, McCaughan (1985) maintained that "the adolescent therapist's response to the clinical setting often parallels the delinquent's
reaction to the structure of the therapeutic milieu" (p. 415). Feeling
unappreciated and misused by a situation so dedicated to external
controls, the therapist may readily empathize with the disturbed
adolescent's experience of being victimized.

For me, the notions of a split social field and parallel process went
hand in hand. The former interpreted the patient's acting out as a
response to milieu conflicts; the latter interpreted the therapist's
acting out as a function of feeling at odds with superiors. As a
consequence, countertransference again became redefined for me.
No longer simply intrapsychic, a matter of unresolved conflicts, as
explained by Masterson, neither was it narrowly interpersonal, a
question of feelings that a patient had "put into" his therapist, as
suggested by projective identification. Rather, both patient and
therapist were answering essential ambiguities in their situations by
their actions. While their personal styles and temperaments were
certainly relevant to the particular actions each took, a full account
of the conduct of each had to include the context that had set it in
motion (see McCaughan, 1985, p. 424).

Once given this key with which I could compare my own and Kay's
experiences, I saw instances of it everywhere. First and foremost, I
began to identify how my problematic relationship with my supervisor paralleled and, in effect, communicated (if essentially nonverb-
ally) my troublesome relationship with my patient. Just as Kay was
berating me for the unfairness of her hospitalization, so too was I
complaining to my supervisor about what I experienced as the unit's
unfairness to me. My conduct in supervision, in other words, demonstrated for my supervisor how Kay overpowered and made me
anxious. I "told" him what transpired by identifying with and then
reenacting how Kay acted with me. My supervisor's response to my

increasingly shrill demands that he *do* something seemed also to mirror my reactions to Kay. While he insisted that I maintain a fairly narrow focus on the patient-therapist dyad, I complied with my concentration on projective identification. In sum, my supervisor and I both ran away from what we experienced as the other's unreasonable expectations with some version of a flight into therapy. We gained short-term (if shortsighted) relief from what nagged at us by limiting our gaze.

By thus viewing these two ostensibly separate relationships as, in fact, one multidirectional network, I was able to make explicit and reflect upon the "conversation" between them. Not incidentally, I was also able to empathize with what I imagined to be my supervisor's experience, thereby ameliorating, to some extent, my fears that our differences might be irremediable. Optimally, of course, I would have had an in-house supervisor who could have responded more directly to my interests and practical needs. By lessening my tendency to displace all my frustrations with Kay and the team onto him, though, I grew better able to appreciate the clinical advice he could offer.

The reconsiderations engendered by a systemic perspective also relaxed my defensive need to think of the milieu as all wrong and of myself as all right. Because my own acting out on the unit no longer carried with it a conviction of my inadequacy as a psychotherapist, I was freer to examine how it, too, was an expression of a multidirectional network. Equipped with the concepts of parallel process and the split social field, I could look back on and make new sense of two occasions, described in the following paragraphs, when I had made important treatment decisions without consulting the team.

In early December I increased Kay's sessions with me from three to four a week. Reacting to the ultimatum that the team had just handed her at the special meeting, I reasoned that if we were demanding that she demonstrate her commitment to our program, the least I could do would be to redouble my commitment to her. After all, there was no explicit rule that therapists could not arrange sessions according to the specific needs of the patients, and even my supervisor had remarked on Kay's articulateness and potential for using insight-oriented psychotherapy. What is more, a peer of mine had been seeing one of her patients four times a week since the summer; if she could take such liberties, then surely so could I.

Let me be clear. Even now, I think that increasing the frequency and length of Kay's sessions could have benefited her treatment. The problems arose because I made this important decision on my own, as if I could circumvent the team and its need for a mutually agreed-upon and coordinated plan. I do not recall deciding consciously to hide Kay's additional weekly session, but I certainly failed to record the change anywhere, even in my personal notes. I vaguely remember casually informing my supervisor at our next meeting and his expressing mild concern that I bring the matter up at the next team meeting.

If I had any illusion that my isolation could shield my secret from the milieu's observation, however, it promptly shattered at the December 11 team meeting. In a confrontation that confirmed my sense that it was "me against them," the team sternly asked me to reflect on the significance of what I had done. All I could hear of their opinion was that I had "overidentified" with my patient, a charge against which I adamantly defended myself.

The standoff continued for another week. I saw Kay four times, in apparent defiance of everyone. I do not remember if anyone said anything at the December 18 team meeting, although in my notes I wrote that there was another very heated discussion about whether Kay "had fulfilled her part of the contract." This team meeting immediately preceded another special meeting, this time with CAS, to inform them of what we would say about Kay at her next court appearence two days hence. After a few negotiations, the team agreed to keep her hospitalized until her next review, scheduled tentatively for February. I felt disgruntled that we were not willing to make a longer-term commitment, but kept my own counsel at this conference with "outsiders."[8]

Later the same day, as I was meeting with another patient in the unit's day area, my team leader interrupted us and insisted that she needed to say something immediately. She told me that I was to resume seeing Kay three times a week by the first of the year. She would tolerate no further arguments; I would do what I was told to

---

[8] Ironically, the note that I wrote on this meeting for Kay's chart concluded with Team B's request that CAS assign only *one* CAS worker to her case from the several whom we had met. While it was certainly true, as I remarked, that "it [was] confusing and countertherapeutic to have so many workers involved," my observation about CAS likely expressed my anger at my team members for similar reasons: I experienced their involvement in Kay's treatment as also confusing and countertherapeutic interference and wished that they would assign me a more autonomous role.

do. At this lowest of low points during my training at State, I felt treated like a child and, even worse, a criminal. Instead of being praised for my best efforts, I was subjected to unfair rebukes.[9]

Looking back on all this from the perspective of the milieu literature that I was reading, I was impressed first by the parallels between Kay's protestations and my own. My acting out and subsequent ultimatum from the team leader had recapitulated the situation that my patient was in. Kay, too, had flaunted the unit rules egregiously, by running away, in response to which she received an unforgiving ultimatum: she either had to commit herself to working with the team, or she would have to seek treatment someplace else. As a consequence, both Kay and I felt unfairly accused and frustrated that the unit refused to acknowledge all the good work we had done. Generally, we experienced the team as unsympathetic and ourselves as trapped and humiliated by its unreasonable demands.

Analogous to my relationship with my supervisor, one could interpret my acting out as a nonverbal communication to my colleagues. Instead of talking about how helpless and angry I felt, I was evoking these feelings in them by breaking the rules. By identifying with and acting like my contrary patient, I was telling them, without admitting it openly, about the frustration that she made me feel. From this perspective, their calling the special meeting was an understandable, if less than optimal, answer. Just as I "fled into the therapy" during this period, eschewing a more systemic examination of her treatment in the hospital, so too did team members narrowly focus on Kay's commitment to hospitalization rather than consider their possible contributions to her difficulties on the unit. For myself as well as for the team as a whole, constricting our focus provided some sense that we had regained control of a nearly impossible situation.

Returning to the notion of the split social field allowed me to develop further the parallel communications between Kay, the team,

---

[9] Less than an hour later, the nurse supervisor summoned me to her office. In place of the further chastisement that I expected, however, she asked if I would be willing to accompany Kay to court on Friday. She and the team leader agreed, she said, that I would be better able to speak for the team than Kay's social worker. Feeling an uneasy mix of flattery and manipulation, I reluctantly agreed. Was this an attempt to make me feel more appreciated? Was I being coerced into cohesiveness with a team that I presently despised? Or was it evidence of further splitting between the team's two powers?

and me. In this view, my acting out was not just a communication from me to the staff but my own response to conflicts among them that they were not discussing directly. Certainly, tensions on the unit were particularly high in December, as this exasperated and sarcastic passalong from the evening to the daytime staff clearly attests:

> In the joy of the present unit status, it could be decreased some if the little people could be informed about things. It is smoother for the kids and us if we are told before the patient arrives to the unit, to anticipate their presence, so the room can be prepared, since none of them are ready. In addition, the room we chose had an extremely rank odor which almost caused two evening staff members to need resuscitation. While scrubbing down the room we found the culprit. It seems that whoever found the garbage can that [female patient] had been urinating in elected to place it in [room] 27 to become very ripe and kill someone. *We're supposed to be a 24 hour team, could we please continue working like one* [from 12/11, italics added].

Interestingly, the problem here, as with my team, was an unsettling lack of cohesiveness and coordinated effort. The writer is accusing her colleague(s) of irresponsible conduct and an equally serious failure to provide important information for the smooth functioning of the unit. This suggests that Team B's divisiveness over Kay may have reflected, in part, more broadly based unit dynamics. Kay and I may have been among the unwitting (if not innocent) spokespersons for the system's distress.

A similar, although less acrimonious, network of parallel phenomena culminated three months later in my allowing Kay to read her chart. In the session that she did so, on March 24, I also noticed that she had pierced a fourth set of holes in her ears some time since our last appointment on March 21. Given how many of the unit's patients had histories of self-destructive behavior, the possession of any sort of sharp instrument, much less cutting oneself in even the most conventional way, was strictly forbidden. Thus, more or less simultaneously, both of us had broken the rules by not consulting first—I with the team and she with the milieu staff—before acting as we did, and the respective authorities soundly scolded both of us when they, in turn, took note of our misdeeds. As significant as the similarities between Kay's and my behavior, however, are those which I can draw between my behavior and the staff's. After a review of the episode, it seems credible to conclude that we, each in our own way, were all reacting to and testing out our fears of being abandoned.

During this period, Kay was feeling vulnerable because her mother was scheduled to have a hysterectomy on March 22. Her terror that her mother would die, which she discussed at length both in and out of her therapy sessions, became exacerbated by her extreme sensitivity to being forsaken.[10] The staff and I agreed to interpret her ear-piercing in light of these recent events, that is, as an act of self-mutilation that expressed to us how fragile and needy she felt.

What Kay most immediately needed was our prompt response to her acting out, but this was not forthcoming. After moaning and groaning and ostentatiously twisting her earrings, she finally succeeded, at least a day after the fact, to get me to look at what she had done. Even though I then told the head nurse (but without writing it down), the staff did not intervene for another day and a half. For all her heartfelt protestations when staff then took all her earrings from her, Kay, and apparently everyone else, soon dropped the issue once we had properly addressed it. In fact, a passalong from three weeks later asks whatever happened to the "earring issue," and it was only after further discussion at that point that staff returned the earrings to Kay, on April 17. It appeared that the assurance that we were looking after her was more important to Kay than the earrings per se.

In my case, I tested how carefully the staff were watching me by writing a passalong three days before I actually showed Kay her chart about how much she had been pressuring me. While I did not say that I intended to satisfy her demands, I certainly left the possibility open. On March 21 I wrote the following:

> Kay has been demanding all week to see her chart (with me). She finally did some work on this, but remained pretty damn hostile! She talked about how confusing and hurtful it is not to be able to figure something out and to feel like no one at State is being direct with her. She also said she wanted help tracking her progress here, to get a different perspective on herself . . . I thought it was good she could let me know how she was feeling.

While Kay was pushing me to tell her directly what we on the staff thought of her, I now think that I was pushing my colleagues to see

---

[10] The symbolic significance of Mrs. Z having a "rotten" womb that she needed to get rid of may have heightened further Kay's sense that there was no place for her in her mother's life.

just how far they would let me go. At some level, I knew that they would not want Kay to see what they had written about her, but I let her nonetheless to make sure that the staff would notice and set limits on my actions. I needed to know, as did Kay, that the team had not abandoned me.

As in the previous example, my acting out mimicked the bind in which I felt Kay had placed me. In this sense, it was a communication to the team about our interpersonal dynamics that I could not yet put into words. This analysis is incomplete, however, because it ignores the significance of the staff's lapses in watchfulness. They, too, were pushing their superiors and implicitly asking to be noticed. Just as Kay feared her mother's loss to a dangerous operation, so too did A-2 staff fear a loss: the promotion of the nurse supervisor to another position within the hospital.

Toward the end of February, State had asked the nurse supervisor to serve as acting nurse administrator for the hospital as a whole. Although the appointment was limited to "about four months," the possibility that she would permanently leave the unit was very real indeed. For better or for worse, this woman provided much of the A-2's direction and cohesiveness. Her consistent guidance was fundamental to the staff's capacity to stay on task. Consequently, the staff felt rudderless and angry when she was absent. At some level, they may have magically hoped that their own acting out would pull her back to their side. To the extent that this was the case, they, like Kay and me, were enacting their sense of being without direction and asking, by their misconduct, to have "mother" rein them in.

The intellectual flexibility that I gained from my reading course (an articulated awareness of viewing my situation from multiple points of view) was in many ways its own reward. The idea that I was a part of a much larger system gave me a perspective on my role that had been sorely lacking before. The milieu gained a meaningful place in my thinking about practicing psychotherapy in a hospital, and I reveled in making sense of interactions that had previously been so much "noise."

The increasing flexibility of my thinking, at first limited to a classroom, gradually extended to my actual relationships on the unit. Not surprisingly, as I exchanged hostility for interest in the multidirectional network of my workplace, the staff appeared to be (and in all probability was) a more likeable group. I included them more often in reflections and conversations about how I could best treat Kay; I enjoyed a sense of belonging and stopped fighting the expectation that I be a team player. This is not to say that all of us lived happily ever after; there continued to be acting out and disagreements all around. But for the concluding four months of my training at State, I was confident that I had a voice that others would seriously listen to, much as the staff and my supervisor were reassured that I would listen to them.

An episode in early June illustrates the practical difference that this improved cohesiveness made: By late spring Kay, no longer considered at risk for elopement, became heavily involved in her discharge planning. While it seemed increasingly unlikely that she would leave the hospital before I did (on June 30), the team was doing everything possible to have her placed by summer's end. Accompanied by a favorite milieu worker, Merry, Kay reportedly did well at an interview for one out-of-state placement on June 2. Back on the unit she was more volatile, but this was easily attributable to her understandable anxiety.

With the change of season and her interviews, Kay wanted to go shopping for new clothes and arranged with another milieu worker, Frances, to take her on June 10. Both the team leader and the nurse supervisor gave their approval. According to a chart note on June 7, Kay "made a point of telling Merry about her plans to go shopping with Frances." Later that weekend, however, Frances had second thoughts and called the unit to say that she was "very uncomfortable with taking Kay shopping." Yet another worker, Daryl, noting the call in a passalong, stated that she would "let Kay know on Monday she won't be going shopping on Tuesday and that Frances will talk to her on Tuesday."

By Monday morning, the situation had escalated. In my notes from June 9 I wrote the following:

> When I arrived on unit 9:15 AM [team leader] pulled me aside saying there were new complications re Kay's shopping pass: Frances (who'd told me Friday that she and Kay'd talked and that they'd be going on pass together) had called unit Saturday eve. after being on unit all day, saying she couldn't take Kay after all. If there were any further details [team leader] did not know them . . . Frances isn't at work today. This AM, [team leader] continues, staff noticed that Kay's walls were "stripped bare." A clear, but unstated assumption was that these 2 events were related: presumably, Frances feared Kay's running from her and, in fact, Kay is stripping her room in preparation for same.

Daryl and [recreational therapist] confronted Kay about [removing] posters and Kay gave some story about making [rock star] collage. [Recreational therapist] later told me that Kay looked depressed—in bad shape. [Team leader] said Kay looked bad and was being assessed for elopement risk. She hadn't yet told her anything about needing follow-up on her abnormal Pap smear [which we had learned on Friday]. All [recreational therapist] could add later in AM was that Kay's "depression" quickly turned to real anger. No one seemed to have *any* clues as to precipitating factors—e.g., a phone call from mother, etc.

Later the same day, in an extensive passalong about Kay's session with me, I commented as follows:

Basically Kay feels hurt and betrayed that F. wasn't clear with her about the shopping pass; knew this had to do with fears she would run. Said it was going to be harder for her to trust again and did some real checking out with me to see if I'd give her honest responses. I checked out her impulses to run and *don't* think ER [elopement risk, the term the unit used for precautions against a patient's running away] is necessary.

Kay informed me during the same session that she had herself received a letter from the gynecologist about her abnormal Pap smear, and the rest of the passalong addressed itself to that. My therapy notes, however, contain more extensive details of our conversation about what had occurred:

[Kay told me that] she and Daryl got into a "shouting match." Kay broke a mirror and was going to cut self. Realized that this would be used to label her "impulsivity," so gave Daryl glass. . . . Good eye contact; wanted acknowledgment for not cutting herself . . . I ask if she talked to her mother over weekend. She startles and says it's none of my business . . . I ask if she knows why we ask. [No.] I explain that her not sleeping, getting upset, etc., often associated with call from her mother. A huffy, "I knew that—I just wanted to see if you'd answer honestly." [Shortly thereafter tells me about letter from gynecologist.]

In a similar conversation with Merry (also recorded in detail), Kay concluded by stating that she felt "invested" in finding a placement and that she'd "reached the point of being able to tell [us when she felt impulsive]." That evening the milieu staff decided that there was no present need to consider her at risk for running away.

I have presented these events at length because I think that they demonstrate the modest but substantial benefits of improved communication and teamwork. Eight months after her admission on A-2, high drama and ambivalence still accompanied working with Kay; she still aroused unexpected and disconcertingly passionate disagreements among us. But in this instance, consistent checking back and forth between all the players, including Kay, circumvented the lasting misunderstandings and recriminations that had characterized earlier interactions. Not only were we all more open and willing to admit to doubts and disappointments, but the assurance that we were working together toward common goals helped us to keep daily crises in perspective.

I introduced this section by alluding to Mahler's concept of rapprochement, a notion I metaphorically applied to the improvements in my relationships to the milieu and the team. Earlier in the year, I had been like a toddler who had just learned to walk; I had rushed away from my superiors as if I had the capacity to do without them. A few tumbles later, I had to relinquish this illusion. Sobered, I modified my practicing as an autonomous psychotherapist to include frequent "refuelings" from those on whom I depended.

My growing identification of myself as a team player, however, did not resolve my difficulties in any absolute sense. As Mahler, among others, frequently pointed out, negotiating autonomy and dependence is a lifelong task. Challenging a too enthusiastic embrace of a milieu perspective, for instance, Harold Searles (1979) argued for the value of a therapist's independence on a psychiatric inpatient unit. He cautioned that "the individual therapist needs to become free of having to campaign, in his work, for the goals the ward milieu sets up as laudable." If the therapist becomes too "reality-bound," Searles explained, he "will be unable to discern all-important symbolic meanings in what the patient . . . is saying" (p. 107).

In concluding this chapter, I will consider the possibly deleterious effects of my increasing valuation of solidarity with the team on Kay's individual psychotherapy. Specifically, I will examine A-2's rituals around patients saying good-byes as an example of a goal that the milieu staff set up as laudable. I will debate whether and to what extent my eventual subscription to this goal expressed *my own* need for a happy ending to my training year and compromised my ability to discern "all-important symbolic meanings" in what Kay was saying.

THE "SAYING GOOD-BYES" RITUAL

Far from a simple matter of an adios at the doorway, saying good-byes on the unit was a lengthy and highly public procedure. Carried out primarily in the thrice-weekly milieu meetings, this ritual was enacted in two practices. First of all, staff expected individual patients who were leaving to articulate to the group what they had gained from and would miss about their various relationships on the unit. Second, when all of the therapists finished their training on the 30th of June, we expected the patients to express again their appreciation. Because for Kay there was an effort to coordinate her leaving with mine, her good-byes combined what typically occurred at two separate times.

While A-2 stressed the importance of good-byes over and over, I do not recall its rationale ever being explained. The strong implicit assumption, however, was that it was for the patients' benefit, that it concerned their need to separate and to come to terms with this trauma. Because we considered separation an essential phase of the treatment, we saw saying good-bye to the milieu as an integral component of this process.

By and large, for individual patients being discharged this unstated argument was plausible. Given all that they had experienced with the staff and their fellow patients, a group-wide review and formal leave-taking seemed justified. In actuality, this rite of passage included a great deal of teasing and chastising and only rarely achieved anything approaching heartfelt conviction. Even so, talking with everyone about what it meant to leave could be viewed as one aspect of an unquestionably significant transition.[11]

By contrast, the psychotherapeutic need for the patients staying

---

[11] As discussed in greater length in Chapter 3, Masterson formally identified separation as the third stage of a borderline adolescent's hospitalization, following an initial period of testing and a longer period of working through. The crucial difference between Masterson's schema and the milieu's unexamined assumptions about good-byes, however, was that the milieu staff did not insist that testing and working through end before separation began. Thus, someone like Kay could catapult from testing to separation with virtually no working through.

on the unit to say good-bye to the departing student therapist group bears scrutiny less well. While losing their individual therapist was unsettling and even deeply disturbing, patients could address this disruption only superficially in a community meeting. Rather, the effect of all the therapists leaving was most pronounced for the staff, who were left behind once again. Having made their peace with these trainees, they would soon face a new group. Particularly because there was neither a traditional ceremony or party to mark the trainees' passage, I think that it was for the staff, in this situation, that the patients said good-byes. The patients were the appointed spokespersons for the milieu, and it was the milieu that profited.

By not directly participating in the saying good-byes ritual, the permanent staff spared themselves a direct confrontation with just how angry and vulnerable the students' exodus made them feel. They focused instead on what the patients suffered and helped the patients to cope. They thereby preserved the alliance with the therapists, which had been so difficult to establish, while simultaneously affirming their own indispensability to the unit. They could joke in the nurses' station about the "mess" the trainees were leaving them without putting at risk the cohesiveness and confidence so central to staff morale.

We students also profited from this indirect communication through the patients as it helped us to surmount whatever guilt we may have felt. In effect, we colluded with the staff in our shared concentration on the adolescents, masking our own ambivalence about leaving with the task we had in common. Thus, even though we *encouraged* patients initially to be distraught, we could then work with the staff to interpret this therapeutically. By supporting the patients as they worked through their issues with separation and loss, we could take their finally saying their good-byes as an affirmation of their getting better and of the good work we had done.[12] Let me now look specifically at how these good-byes affected Kay.

Team B worked long and hard throughout the spring to have Kay discharged by June 30; in fact, we actually discharged her about six

_____

[12] A much more thorough sociological account of the contradictory pressures on psychotherapy trainees and their patients is Ruth Coser's (1979) *Training in Ambiguity: Learning Through Doing in a Mental Hospital.* Complementing her overview, and my discussion of good-byes, is Robert Klein's (1981) "The Patient-Staff Community Meeting: A Tea-Party with the Mad Hatter." The latter focuses on how an inpatient milieu meeting answers the very real, albeit unconscious, needs of the staff.

weeks later. To all intents and purposes, then, her individual good-
byes to the milieu coincided with her group participation in saying
good-byes to the therapists. Superficially, this appeared to simplify
matters for her. Like the trainees, she had presumably gained what
she could from the hospital and, like us, she was leaving. Unlike the
other patients and staff who were staying longer on the unit, she was
not being left behind. Consequently, it seemed to be a shorter and
easier step for her than for the patients who were not ready for
discharge to articulate what she had learned from and would miss
about the milieu as a whole.

This formulation of events, however, assumed that Kay was
psychologically ready to leave. In fact, her discharge date represented a delicate web of negotiations and compromises between
me, the team, and CAS and had little to do with developments in
Kay's individual psychotherapy per se. When discharge planning
began in late February, she had yet to graduate from testing the
unit's sincerity and reliability in working with her; no one was
convinced that she would have worked through her problems adequately by June. We maintained this fiction, however, for two very
different reasons. Pragmatically, the team had to argue that Kay was
sufficiently better in order to persuade residential placements to
consider accepting her. In addition, our willing suspension of disbe-
lief allowed me to cooperate with my teammates, thereby enabling
the team to remain united in their dealings with CAS.[13]

A number of factors influenced my initial decision to stop fighting
the team about Kay's continuing need for hospitalization. First and
foremost was what I got in return: a tacit agreement that they would
no longer label her untreatable and that we would seriously look for
the best placement for her. By February I was familiar enough with
discharge proceedings to know that they could easily occupy several
months. At the very least, therefore, I could count on Kay remaining
on A-2 for about as long as I would; I would not lose my patient
before I myself left.

I used a version of the milieu literature to support my change of
heart, reasoning that it was countertherapeutic to maintain a "split

---

[13] As human behavior is impossible to predict, it is quite possible that Kay
succeeded in the residential placement she went to from State. My point here,
though, is that the team was not primarily concerned with assessing her psychopathology but, rather, with negotiating the institutional and political complexities of
getting her discharged.

social field." In many respects, this argument was valid; Kay certainly benefited from an awareness that her caretakers were not fighting. The laudable cloak of team cohesiveness and collaboration, though, may have hidden my more selfish motivations for wanting to belong to the team. Weary of the dissension that had made me feel so split off, I was happy to have good reasons for letting it go. I blurred important distinctions to strengthen my newly adopted position and conveniently conflated the dangers of covert disagreements with a legitimate advocacy of my individual work with Kay.

Finding a good place that would have Kay promised to be arduous, and this practical consideration further enhanced my willingness to begin discharge planning in February. As Kay herself once bitterly remarked, her history made her undesirable; who would want an oppositional prostitute-molester? Additionally, most residential settings preferred younger adolescents, and, for legal reasons if nothing else, Kay would need a placement that could keep her until she was 21. Last but not least was the fact that she was a ward of the state, and CAS had their own rules about what institutions they would fund.

Successfully placing my patient was more tangible and immediately satisfying than the elusive goals of individual psychotherapy. Challenged by the difficulty of getting different groups together, I liked the sense that I was important in bringing this about. As much as I complained about calling placements, writing reports, and accompanying Kay three times to court, I enjoyed feeling recognized for what I was doing. I quieted my doubts about my effectiveness as a clinician with evidence of my increasing effectiveness as a member of the team. The question is whether and to what extent this compromised my work with Kay.

With newly established harmony, the team shifted from insisting on Kay's commitment to the program to our shared concentration on getting her out. As a result, she had scarcely begun to settle down on the unit before we began to pressure her to say her good-byes. This shift was immediately reflected in my construction of the case, as is apparent from two succeeding chart notes that I wrote on February 13 and 28. In the first, I made the following observations:

> The past two weeks have been turbulent, but not unproductive for the patient. While she continues to complain about the unit, she has also

expressed an increased willingness to try to "work." She has also brought up how she has already "changed" and more openly expresses her longing to be connected and cared for by members of the staff.

In this note I emphasized how well Kay was "working" and making connections with the milieu staff. In anticipation of her case review on February 24, I was still campaigning for how she could profit from continuing hospitalization. By contrast, having agreed with the team and CAS on the merits of discharging her in the summer, my next note anticipated the difficulties of dealing with her "abandonment depression":

Over the past two weeks the patient has been increasingly anxious about her treatment plan, the possibility of discharge planning, and her progress review in court on 2/28. Her mood is more labile than it has been for quite some time, fluctuating within a single session from sullenness to hostility to cooperative conversation to giddy overexcitement. Given the patient's history of abandonment, which she now sets up to be repeated over and over again, coupled with her defensive need to appear mature, one can only imagine the intensity of her apprehension. Along with this, the patient alternates between experiencing her therapist as a trustworthy ally and as a traitor, another caretaker who has let her down.

No longer did I present Kay as being at the threshold of the working through stage; from here on out, the requirements of termination dominated her treatment.

Throughout this period I battled the worrisome possibility that Kay had made a realistic appraisal of my inconsistencies and that I was truly more traitor than ally. Rather than explore this extensively in our individual sessions, however, I hid my doubts behind an interpretation of her psychopathology. A language of abandonment and loss was useful in this situation; it enabled me to describe her distress while remaining conveniently noncommittal about its sources. I could portray the terrible time Kay was having in saying good-byes without either seriously challenging the discharge plan or questioning how my involvement in carrying it out might have been interfering with the psychotherapy. What is more, because the team and milieu staff were familiar with this way of talking, it reaffirmed our still fragile sense that we were working together.

Despite the gaps in my attention to what she was telling me, Kay was persistent in her efforts to get me to listen. Predictably, she was herself ambivalent about her future. At one moment she wanted nothing better than to get out of the hospital; she had said from the start that she did not belong there. At other times, though, when she felt unwanted and homeless, she tried hard to let us know that she thought our decision stank.

On at least four separate occasions in the late winter and spring, Kay immediately followed talk about her discharge from A-2 with complaints of a "foul-smelling discharge" from her vagina. On February 26, for example, Merry wrote the following note in Kay's chart:

> Given information that discharge planning is going on and [Kay] seemed upset. Complained of a vaginal discharge with odor and yellowish color and the doctor was notified.

A similar note by the team leader was recorded on March 18, followed by another (longer) one from Merry on March 21:

> Our conversation covered several of her current issues. She seems to be feeling really bad that her father never provided her with the necessary nurturance she felt she needed, nor any other type of support (monetary). . . . In her room she was crying and got in touch with the type of qualities she would like to have in the men she attracted—intelligent, educated, snazzy dresser, sensitive. . . . Talked about her [elopement risk status] and how it's never acknowledged to her that she's making progress. Earlier complained about vaginal discharge and a very foul odor.

Not only did I not pursue "all-important symbolic meanings" in similar complaints that Kay made to me, but I at one point recommended that she start wearing cotton underwear! In other words, I remained steadfastly "reality-bound," taking care, with the staff, of her physical needs while ignoring their possible psychological significance.

Patient good-byes to the therapists, which commenced in mid-April, only obscured further what leaving State meant to Kay. Coupled with my interpretation of her "abandonment depression," they shielded me further from dealing as honestly as I might have with her legitimate reasons for being angry at going. One example will suffice.

It was a truism among the staff on A-2 that for the patients "getting angry is easier than saying good-bye." Eventually, we assumed confidently, they would come around to admitting their attachments to us. For the staff, instead, I think that the opposite was true: it was far easier for us to say how we cared than to admit that anger might be appropriate. We avoided direct confrontations with our patients' expressions of it by neatly and quickly interpreting them away.

During a session on May 2, for instance, when she was "berating everything," Kay proceeded to complain bitterly about my being "just a student":

> Particularly adamant about not wanting to be an experimental rat, a lab rat. I'm just a student and she wants to be seen by someone with *years* of experience. She talked to her Dad and he said he thought I was full of BS—[he] knew she'd change back as soon as she left State [into] an impulsive, loudmouthed teenager. [Kay went on to say that] she could've done all changes on her own *without* us. [She thinks that] I can't imagine how awful it is to be at this roach motel. I have a decent family, my parents are probably still together, they supported me, at least emotionally, etc. Degrades me personally and psychology generally. Generally makes me feel shut out. But doesn't leave.

In the subsequent team meeting when this session was discussed, I ascribed Kay's devaluing of me as "her present strategy" for coping with our imminent separation. As she could not risk admitting feeling connected to me openly, I maintained, she covered her sorrow at my leaving with her own angry rejection. By going no further than the unit's tried-and-true interpretation, I supported their needs more than hers with respect to saying good-byes.

This is not to say that this formulation had no merit, just that it stopped short of a full analysis of what Kay was telling me. As I review it now, two related themes seem to have warranted more exploration. First, she wanted a therapist "with *years* of experience" precisely because, unlike student therapists, they stayed around. In effect, she *had* been an experiment in my learning to practice psychotherapy; when I was finished with my training I would leave, irrespective of whether or not she had herself left. Second, my exclusive focus on the extent to which Kay degraded me missed entirely her longing to have a life like mine, complete with loving parents who were "probably still together." Given this gap between our experiences, she despaired of my ever imagining hers. Ironically, given my usual sensitivity to countertransference, in the therapy note I described feeling shut out and anxious about *Kay's* leaving before that session ended without reflecting on the insight this might have yielded about her.

I can debate but not resolve the drawbacks of a milieu perspective for practicing psychotherapy on an inpatient unit. All in all, though, I think it was the most comprehensive viewpoint on my various relationships in the hospital and on ways of thinking and talking about my work with Kay. Without excluding what was useful about the theories of projective identification and the borderline, it best allowed me to "converse" with a problematic situation while holding myself open to that situation's "back talk." Nonetheless, it, like any other theoretical design, could not satisfactorily address every aspect of what I did. In concluding this case study, I return in the following chapter to Schön's paradigm of the "reflective practitioner" and explore more generally its relevance for the practice of psychoanalytic psychotherapy.

6

CONVERSATION

*Taking therapy as it is and watching what is done, we
understand in all kinds of ways that the therapist
understands his patient in all kinds of ways, and we
see that each type of understanding employed by a
therapist has its special impact on his patient. And now
it must be noted that understanding the effects of each
type of understanding is itself another form of
therapeutic understanding.*

Lawrence Friedman, *The Anatomy of Psychotherapy*

More than any other training experience, my work at State Psychiatric Hospital, especially with Kay, confronted me with the discrepancies between my preconceived ideas about what is supposed to
happen in clinical practice and the often unanticipated and confusing
events that actually occur. I was at that point completing a third year
of formal class work devoted, in part, to a variety of psychotherapeutic theories or models juxtaposed to diagnostic and therapeutic
practica, which, presumably, would give me an opportunity to apply
what I had learned. Any number of case studies that I had read
strengthened this expectation. By and large, they began by defending
a theoretical position and told a story that demonstrated the correct-
ness of their point of view. Critical enough to doubt the equal validity
of all such theories and illustrations, I nonetheless believed, as

Lawrence Friedman (1982) wryly observed of psychoanalytic psychotherapists generally, that, "unlike every other long-term relationship, treatment has a neat, planned structure" (p. 18).

The actuality of working with Kay was anything but neatly
planned. Instead, it was, by turns, noisy, conflictual, magical, and
only occasionally well-coordinated. Even as it became more reliably
a collaborative endeavor with my patient and my colleagues, each of
our motivations remained complicated, and the results of our
common effort unpredictable. The experience was unlike anything
my education had taught me to expect.

My problem was not just the practical confusion that Kay generated about what I should do and say from moment to moment in our
relationship. To some extent I felt prepared to learn about such
things as the proper timing of interpretations and the judicious use
of self-disclosure. What unsettled me far more was the helpless
feeling that I did not know how to think about what I was doing.
Diagnoses, treatment plans, and therapeutic technique—concepts
that, in the classroom, had promised to guide me—seemed vacuous
and meaningless once I became immersed in an apparently hostile
milieu with an indisputably hostile patient.

Even the clinical theories of interpersonalist psychoanalysts,
such as Harry Stack Sullivan, which I had studied so carefully and
enthusiastically, failed to assuage my despair at the flimsiness and
fickleness of my own understanding. Although Sullivan (1954) described the therapist's stance as that of a "participant observer" and
argued for there being "no psychiatric data that can be observed
from a detached position by a person in no way involved in the
operation" (p. 57), what he wrote suggested that he remained
unruffled by what such involvement might entail. Increasingly, I was
convinced that no published case study resembled in the slightest
my own distressingly blind efforts. Even worse, I was embarrassed to
find myself relying on theorists, such as Masterson, who in asserting
the objective and logical application of therapeutic procedures
adopted a position antithetical to the one I had thought I believed in.

My dismay deepened before it abated; a chasm yawned between
my understanding and what was happening. I, who so treasured
ideas, was using them haphazardly, too rattled and pressured to
reflect on their implications. Far from flying by the seat of my pants,
I felt dragged over a painfully bumpy course by forces, from both
within and without, that were beyond my control.

Reading Donald Schön's (1983) *The Reflective Practitioner* in the midst of my practicum helped me to right myself. At the time, his articulation of "how professionals think in action" gave me a way of comprehending my seemingly disparate attempts to apply diverse theories as a continuing "conversation" with my "indeterminate situation." By loosening my expectations about how a set of ideas or theoretical principles could guide my psychotherapy, he revitalized my badly shaken faith in the relevance of my reading and course work and initiated an ongoing series of reflections on how I might actually use theory in my clinical practice. Not insignificantly, reading Schön also suggested the organization of this case study: the threading together of three theoretically distinct concepts—the borderline adolescent, projective identification, and the milieu—into an account of my increasingly self-aware "thinking-in-action" as I interacted with Kay.

In *Educating the Reflective Practitioner* (1987), Schön argued that "professional education should be redesigned to combine the teaching of applied science with coaching in the artistry of reflection-in-action" (p. xii). Reviewing architectural design, his earlier proto-type for "research in a practice context," he explored how it also provides a model for how educators can foster more systematically the process of construction and discovery essential to converting indeterminate situations into relatively more determinate ones. He proposed that students would profit most from apprenticeships to "master craftsmen," within reflective practica, who

> emphasize surfacing private attributions for public testing, giving direct observational data for one's judgments, revealing the private dilemmas with which one is grappling, actively exploring the other's meaning, and inviting the other's confrontation with one's own [p. 141].

Looking specifically at Sachs and Shapiro's (1974, 1976) use of parallel process in the supervision of psychoanalytic psychotherapy, Schön (1987) argued that the interaction between teacher and student resembles fundamentally the problematic "communication across divergent worlds" between therapist and patient (p. 231). Through conversation about the treatment, supervisors demon-strate to students their own reasoning, uncertainties, and feelings as

they "grope their way for answers" (p. 248), as a means of encouraging students to recognize and participate in the kind of thinking-
in-action basic to the therapeutic process itself. The supervisor
self-consciously uses his or her interactions with the trainee as a
privileged example of the kind of activity the trainee is practicing.

Surprisingly, given his reliance on a wide variety of annotated
transcripts of supervisory sessions to make his argument, Schön
failed to appreciate the didactic power of reading about a professional's struggle to make sense of what often seems an unpredictable
and impossibly complicated relationship. By contrast, I contend
that, like certain kinds of coaching, a case study can model a more
or less disciplined use of theoretical concepts, not as statements of
fact or truth, but as ways of orienting oneself, providing a direction
for one's thinking, and seeing possibilities for understanding and
intervention. Written accounts of clinical practice can demonstrate
a "conversation with uncertainty" in a way that engages their
readers in the same sort of "problem-framing, on-the-spot experiment, detection of consequences and implications, backtalk and
response to backtalk" as does an apprenticeship (Schön, 1987,
p. 158).[1]

---

[1] In 1978, at the University of Chicago, I took a course entitled Rhetoric from David
Smigelskis, an associate professor who teaches both in the College and in the
humanities graduate program of Ideas and Methods. Taking Aristotle's *Rhetoric* as his
starting point, Smigelskis developed a notion of "innovative disciplines" or those
enterprises "which allow one to make more determinate what is relatively indeterminate" (classroom communication, October, 1978). Abstractly stated, the class concerned itself with practical knowledge and the problems inherent in locating oneself
within the same ongoing and open-ended activity that one strives to understand (as
opposed, at least classically, to theoretical knowledge or pure science). Needless to
say, very little could be said at such an abstract level.

In psychotherapy, as in other professional pursuits, Smigelskis maintained, becoming aware of and articulating what one actually is doing (and perhaps not so well)
may enable one to do it better and with greater self-control. As illustrative of this
process, he included among the variety of texts we read, from literary criticism to the
philosophy of science, Harry Stack Sullivan's *The Psychiatric Interview* (1954). We
approached this work not as a "how-to" manual, but as a systematic but far from fixed
framework for developing a flexible understanding of a patient and how he might be
helped.

In many ways, I credit Smigelskis for instilling in me an extremely useful attitude
toward psychotherapeutic practicing that is very consistent with Schön's notion of
"reflection-in-action." Certainly, I share the aim for my case study that Smigelskis set
for his class. In writing about the back-and-forth between understanding and "back
talk" in the specific terms of Kay's treatment, I hope to encourage by my own example
a conversation with uncertainty that I consider basic to the psychotherapeutic task.

In this chapter I develop further my claim for the pedagogical value of reading—and writing—a case study framed as a "conversation with uncertainty." In doing so, I am extending Schön's characterization of "reflection-in-action" to argue that a case study best captures the inherently contextual and self-reflexive qualities of psychotherapeutic knowing. Whereas many case studies convey a sense of initial mystery and discovery, I have rarely read one that focuses more on the ongoing process of "figuring out" than on the solutions such hypotheses yield.[2] Revising our expectations about a case study's rhetoric, role, and function could contribute importantly, I think, to how psychotherapists think about their professional identity and expertise. By my own example, I hope to encourage other psychoanalytic psychotherapists to write similar case studies that make explicit the essentially unpredictable yet indissolubly linked efforts of understanding their patients and themselves.

Thus far, I have used a number of actual and metaphorical conversations to frame my case, conversations with my patient and the hospital milieu, my supervisors, clinical ideas I found ready to use, and with Schön's epistemology of professional practice. Now I will develop my reflections on case studies per se through a similar, if higher order, "conversation" with Irwin Hoffman and Lawrence Friedman, two clinical theorists who also grapple with the essential indeterminacy of the psychotherapeutic relationship and how best to conceptualize psychotherapeutic work. As before, I will not pretend to provide a comprehensive literature review. Edgar Levenson's emphasis on the therapist's "ability to be trapped, immersed, and participating in a system and then to work his way out" (1972, p. 174, see also 1982); Merton Gill's consideration of the "real" relationship be-

---

[2] This is not to say, of course, that mine is the first or only case presentation that acknowledges the therapist's experience of uncertainty and ongoing effort to gain greater clarity. For the most part, though, writers focus either on the experiencing or on the achievement of understanding, not on the dialectic between the two. In recent years, for example, discussions of countertransference have become very prevalent, including Searles (1979) vivid evocations of working with severely disturbed patients. As much as I value such therapeutic portraits, Searles does not examine, as I do, the role *ideas* played both in his constructions of and extrications from clinical situations. At the other end of the spectrum, Kohut (1979), in describing the two analyses of Mr. Z, clearly stated the different implications of his different theoretical commitments but did not use his case to demonstrate how his ideas changed in response to the nitty-gritty of his work. By contrast, my aim in this case is to capture the give-and-take of experiencing and understanding as it unfolded in the specific terms of Kay's psychotherapy.

tween therapist and patient (1983, 1985); Stephen Mitchell's relational concept of the "embedded" analyst (1988); and Donnel Stern's
notion of the therapist "courting surprise" (1990, 1991) are among
other psychoanalytic points of view that helped me to understand
psychotherapy as an inherently open-ended inquiry. In these concluding reflections I wish only to convey the continuing give-and-take
of my ideas with those of others, as I make more determinate the
implications of writing a case study such as this one.

PARTICIPANT OBSERVATION AND THE "BACK TALK" OF IDEAS

Participant observation has haunted the edges of this case study as
an admirable but seemingly unrealizable therapeutic stance. Ironically, as I now reflect on what I have written, the case seems an
unmistakable evocation of this elusive concept. Indeed, Schön
(1983) himself provided a general definition, easily adaptable to the
psychotherapeutic situation, when he wrote that "through his trans-
action with the situation [the practitioner] shapes it and makes
himself a part of it. Hence the sense he makes of the situation must
include his own contribution to it" (p. 163). In effect, in writing my
case, I used Schön's notion of "reflection-in-action" to describe my
ongoing struggle to observe and make sense of my participation
with Kay, by considering my own needs and motivations as well as
hers. In the following pages I draw on Irwin Hoffman's (1983, 1990,
1991) development of a social conception of the patient-therapist
relationship to say more definitively what I mean by participant
observation and how I think case studies can capture and convey its
truly interactive quality.

Hoffman (1991) defined the *social-constructivist* paradigm in
terms of two fundamental propositions: the psychoanalyst inevitably participates in and is influenced by the psychoanalytic relationship, and both patient and analyst actively construct the
meaning of their interactions. Committed to the premise that "the
analyst's understanding is always a function of his or her perspective
at the moment" (p. 77), Hoffman contrasted what amounts to a new
epistemology of practice to more positivistic assumptions of analytic objectivity and the existence of preexisting truths. Far from
having privileged insight into the correct understanding of clinical
phenomena, the analyst, in Hoffman's view, must accept that unfor-

mulated experience is "intrinsically ambiguous and open to a range of compelling interpretations and explications," including those offered by the patient.

In his initially brief but excellent exposition of the social-constructivist paradigm, Hoffman (1983) began with a "radical critique" of two enduring fictions in psychoanalysis: the notion of the analyst as a blank screen and what Hoffman terms the "naive patient fallacy." Locating himself in a long tradition of theorists similarly dissatisfied with the assertion that the patient projects his intrapsychic fantasies and wishes onto an opaque and essentially impersonal clinician, Hoffman distinguished his argument by maintaining that psychoanalysis implies a relationship in the fullest sense. Not only do patients respond to real qualities in their therapists, he argued, but they exert a real and frequently unpredictable effect as well. What is more, like their therapists, patients astutely watch for hidden meanings and conflicts, often interpreting the behavior of their therapists more trenchantly than the therapists themselves (p. 410).

For Hoffman, the analyst's participant observation precludes any conviction that he can see the treatment situation more accurately than the person whom he treats. He does not possess a privileged perspective from which he can differentiate the analysand's idiosyncratic or distorted perceptions from those that are realistic or objective. This is not to say that patients' constructions of the analytic relationship cannot be skewed or limited or self-defeating; obviously they often are. Rather, Hoffman stressed the constraints of the analyst's own personality or countertransference on what he discerns. The reality of patients' thoughts, feelings, and perceptions cannot be divorced from particular situations; likewise, therapists create and discover themselves in their own experiences, including their relationships with their patients.

Extending his earlier work with Gill (1982), Hoffman recast psychotherapeutic expertise and objectivity in terms of the analyst's willingness to bring to light and validate unspoken assumptions and observations. Instead of simply repeating well-established patterns of interaction, the analyst engages the patient in a collaborative inquiry into *each* of their contributions to the therapeutic relationship. Far from objective in the sense of uncovering a preexisting truth, such an investigation nonetheless legitimates the patient's experience of the here-and-now encounter.

By encouraging the patient to voice his perceptions of the analyst and assuming their plausibility as interpretations, the analyst offers the patient a new kind of experience. As Hoffman (1983) put it:

> In this other experience, the patient comes to know that the analyst is not so consumed or threatened by the countertransference that he is no longer able to interpret the transference. For to be able to interpret the transference fully means interpreting, and in some measure being receptive to, the patient's interpretations of the countertransference (Racker, 1968, p.131). What ensues is a subtle kind of rectification. The patient is, in some measure, freed of an unconscious sense of obligation to resist interpreting the analyst's experience in order to accommodate a reciprocal resistance in the analyst [p. 414].

Optimally, the analyst's articulation of a "transference-counter-transference enactment" identifies the patient's perception as only one of several possible scenarios, thereby loosening the patient's sense of its inevitability. By the same token, by taking seriously their patient's point of view about them, analysts can observe and modify their own participation in the psychotherapeutic process.

In his most recent formulation of the social-constructivist paradigm, Hoffman (1991) explicitly related it to Schön's view of professional practice as "reflection-in-action" (p. 79), while underscoring the complexity of "back talk" for a psychotherapist's "conversation with uncertainty." Like the clinician, the patient also endeavors to make sense of an indeterminate situation, trying out various hypotheses about himself, his therapist, and the progress of the treatment.

For example, Kay's rejection of my implicit equating of her crying with "good therapy" had several possible meanings. At the very least, she challenged my application of Masterson's theory, "interpreted" my discomfort with her aggression and enthusiasms, and conveyed her own distress at feeling sad. Whatever its precise significance, Kay "reflected-in-action." In contrast to a landscape, which reveals to an architect the limits and possibilities of his designing, Kay's "back talk" included her own experimental efforts as well as her responses to mine.

Hoffman's conception of participant observation describes a fundamental attitude toward patients and clinical practice and offers a peculiarly psychoanalytic perspective on conversing with uncertainty. Despite my affinity for his social-constructivist paradigm, though, we have chosen dramatically differing ways to write about psychotherapeutic interactions. In part, this reflects differences in our level of analysis: I aim to capture the experience of a particular treatment, while Hoffman tries to work out an epistemology of psychoanalytic understanding. Hoffman, moreover, concerns himself more exclusively with traditional psychoanalysis whereas my interest is in psychoanalytic psychotherapy. In a real sense, however, our choice of rhetoric masks a significant difference in how we think about using theory in practice, with implications for what we consider most important for therapists-in-training to learn.

Hoffman pays scrupulous attention to how psychoanalytic theorists write. Convinced that clinical theory has real consequences for practice, he carefully assesses seemingly slight differences of emphasis and locution for their implicit assumptions about patients and therapists. Specifically, he contends that to be clinically useful, a psychotherapeutic model must foster a radically interpersonal notion of participant observation. Such a model would, in his view,

> encourage the analyst to expect to be caught up in complex patterns of interaction involving ambiguous integrations of repetition and new experience. Similarly, it [would] encourage analysts to expect that their own understanding will inevitably be skewed by their personal participation in the process [1991, p. 81].

Hoffman strongly criticizes a number of allegedly relational theories, in addition to more conservative psychoanalytic viewpoints, for perpetuating a mistaken notion of psychotherapeutic expertise, to the detriment of effective psychotherapeutic treatment.

I do not question Hoffman's aims but want to recommend a different path to their realization. Reflecting on my own training, as I have in this case, convinced me that no theoretical formulation, however sophisticated and experience-near, could sufficiently encourage the clinical goals that, with Hoffman, I endorse. Without minimizing the importance of rigorous conceptualization as an end in itself, I think that a close examination of the different roles that ideas play in a particular therapeutic relationship makes more accessible the "ambiguous integrations of repetition and new experience" that inhere in that relationship.

In other words, I dispute the pedagogical and clinical need to repudiate any and all nonconstructivist theories. Rather, I maintain that the term participant observation embraces any number of theoretical perspectives that the therapist weaves into his evolving understanding of the case. Let me elaborate what I mean in terms of my narrative about working with Kay.

Masterson's model for treating the borderline adolescent falls well outside the boundaries of a constructivist paradigm. Despite his allegiance to object relations theorists, Masterson does not conceive of the patient-therapist interaction as mutually defining and collaborative. Masterson's therapist does not believe that his view of his patients is necessarily skewed by his "personal participation in the process," nor does he alter his interpretations in light of his patients' views of him. Rather, Masterson describes a therapist capable of incisive diagnoses and treatment, who identifies his patients' illnesses and then prescribes a cure. As a theorist, then, Masterson does not encourage the therapist's humility in the face of ambiguity and the revelatory meanings of his patients' interpretations.

I have already criticized Masterson's implicit conceptualization of the therapeutic relationship, for many of the reasons Hoffman presumably would too. Only to criticize his asymmetrical vision of the patient's and therapist's roles, however, would miss entirely the constructive use to which I put it in my actual engagement with Kay. As a novice in overwhelmingly unfamiliar territory, I desperately needed to begin with a discipline, a sense of purpose, and some set of ascertainable goals. This is not to say that another theory might not have answered my needs as well as or better than Masterson's. Rather, my point is that at that early point in my training, I could not sustain the continuous sense of ambiguity and openness that Hoffman advocates without risking complete immobility.

What began as my search for right answers, however, provided me with sufficient confidence as a clinician that I could start to imagine the excitement of an open-ended "conversation with uncertainty." My early adherence to Masterson's prescriptions ended with an appreciation for how I could use Masterson's ideas and treatment plan hypothetically, to construct possible meanings for my interactions with Kay. For this reason, I would include within a constructivist perspective the psychotherapist's use of positions, such as Masterson's, as sources of plausible, if not absolute, interpretations of clinical encounters.

I embraced projective identification for somewhat different motives: to justify, without denying, the strength of my countertransference. Discomforted by my wish to run away from my patient and my anger at the team, I translated my feelings into communications from Kay. I essentially disclaimed responsibility for my emotions by assuming they were hers; I was merely a container for *her* split-off and unmanageable passions.

Hoffman (1983) specifically criticized those Kleinian theorists, such as Bion and Heimann, who describe projective identification with hyperbolic flourish (p. 412). I agree with his judgment that such formulations simply exchange the "blank screen" for an "empty container," thereby retaining an asocial conception of the therapeutic relationship. By contrast, Hoffman classifies Sandler's (1976) more temperate discussion of the analyst's "role responsiveness" within his constructivist paradigm for accepting matter-of-factly that patients will have—and will know that they have—a real effect on their therapist.

Again, I have no quarrel with Hoffman's critique at the level of theory. If anything, I think that the therapist as empty container sounds even less plausible than the therapist as blank screen. Yet the fact remains that at that moment in my treatment of Kay I reveled in this magical notion. The hyperbolic language of the Kleinians captured the emotional tone of my experience far more accurately than drier accounts. Put succinctly, projective identification, with its vivid descriptions and validation of the therapist's emotional involvement with his patient, enabled me to feel less isolated and disturbed by my own tumultuous feelings and thus to persist in observing my participation with Kay. However, what began as a sort of magic trick—interpreting my internal state as a communication from my patient—laid the groundwork for more balanced reflections on the give-and-take of our interactions.

Imagining his conversation with the so-called milieu theorists raises my most serious and far-reaching criticisms of Hoffman's approach. Stanton and Schwartz (1954), the authors of *The Mental Hospital*, descended directly from Sullivan and aligned themselves explicitly with an interpersonalist point of view. Like Hoffman, they placed therapists squarely within the situation they are trying to affect, analyzing how various relationships and tensions shape their understanding and their sense of what they can accomplish. My experience at State convinced me of the utility of this perspective: an essential challenge of working with Kay was becoming aware of the many ways that I might be responding to a multidirectional network. By contrast, Hoffman's discussion of the social-constructivist paradigm does not explore the room it makes for this sort of complexity. For all his insistence on the ambiguity and relativity of patient-therapist interactions, Hoffman limits his scope to a two-person encounter.

More important, Hoffman's paradigm does not account sufficiently for my contention that ideas *always* mediate therapists' ongoing observations of their participation with their patients. For example, a more effective critique of the blank screen than Hoffman offers would invite clinicians to reflect-in-action on why they themselves are using the concept. Several possibilities spring to mind: therapists' defensive need to presume they are in control of the treatment; their wish to identify themselves with Freudian tradition; or the profession's need to establish for other contemporary behavioral scientists that it, too, is an objective and thus credible enterprise. Instead, while Hoffman marvels at the perverse resiliency of this problematic concept, his exclusively dyadic focus constrains an exploration of what fuels its persistence.

Hoffman has every right, of course, to concentrate on traditional psychoanalysis, which obviously differs greatly from inpatient treatment. And yet, even an analysis must contend with a "babble of voices," an indefinitely extended context that surrounds the encounter. This includes not only the analyst's theories and the patient's internalized objects but more sociological forces that limit interpretations and interventions. One need only reflect briefly on the shifting status of psychoanalysis in American culture to realize that what it means just to seek analytic treatment or training is contextually specific. While Hoffman certainly acknowledges this broader notion of the "social construction of reality" (e.g., 1991, p. 95), his paradigm does not go far enough in examining its relevance.

Let me reiterate, though, the main point I am making: Unlike a theory, which, by necessity, must concern itself with internal coherence, a case study like this one exemplifies the "participant-constructivism" that Hoffman proffers. Only a case study—whether written or presented or worked at in supervision—can reflect the multidirectional network between theoretical visions of psychotherapy and what one then sees. It is in viewing how they actually use ideas in practice that clinicians, and especially students, can become aware of what they do. No one theory or set of theories can depict the bumpy course over which we travel with our patients, even those that recognize ambiguity and many sources of meaning. At best, our advocacy of a social-constructivist paradigm can encourage a particular attitude toward our work; it certainly will not predict the perspectives that become implicated in our encounters.

EXPLORING THE SPACES BETWEEN
THEORY AND PRACTICE

Lawrence Friedman also concerns himself with how psychotherapists write. In fact, he began his ambitious account of *The Anatomy of Psychotherapy* (1988) by remarking on the radical disjuncture between the typically confusing complexity of clinical work and its conceptualization:

> Considering that the one thing a therapist knows with assurance is that he is constantly managing tensions between himself and his patient while about everything else he is never sure, the evaporation of this large fact [of the therapist's discomfort] in published accounts is impressive: What therapists know best is least apparent in their writings [p. 5].

It is to Friedman's great credit, however—and to my benefit—that he avoids misleadingly simple exhortations to therapists to just write more plainly. Rather, his book offers a series of meditations on the gap between psychotherapeutic doing and writing that illuminates the multiple, and sometimes conflicting, purposes this disjuncture serves.

In what follows, I summarize my reflective conversation with Friedman's views, beginning with an elucidation of how he sharpened my appreciation for the diverse aims of clinical theory. I then use his penultimate chapter, entitled "Training," as a specific standpoint from which to re-view my thinking about the value of case studies. After summarizing briefly Friedman's suggestions about educating psychotherapists, I consider their relevance to my own account of training. Finally, I further promote case studies as a distinctive means of reflecting that minimizes neither theory nor the unavoidable tensions that therapists feel as they work.

Friedman's unique contribution to an anatomy of psychotherapy stems, I think, from his willingness to preserve the indefinite and troublesome space between therapists' conceptualizations and their practicing in a way that mimics and makes more fruitful the tensions of the work itself. Unlike Hoffman, who concentrates on the formulation of a paradigm per se, Friedman (1988) looks at therapists' paradoxical uses of theory in both creating and obfuscating the therapeutic relationship (p. 514). Thus, in considering further the challenge of clinical writing, Friedman concluded that

> strange as it seems, if we want to talk vividly and specifically about psychotherapy, we cannot just talk plainly. For theory is literally a part of practice; it sits (or hides) in the therapist's mind. Like it or not, theory is half of the doing [p. 9].

Over and over again, through analyses of particular theories, patients' expectations, and the experience of conducting a psychotherapy, Friedman points out how the apparent contradiction between therapeutic actuality and theoretical ideals describes an indeterminateness intrinsic to the psychotherapy itself. On one hand, his book provides brilliant insights into how therapists use theoretical constructs to mask defensively their discomfort with the psychotherapeutic relationship. On the other, however, it shows persuasively the necessity of such "theoretical hallucinations" to clinicians' picturing viable roles for themselves and potentialities for change in their patients (p. 437).

Friedman shares with Schön a fundamental conviction that professional expertise depends upon a genuine commitment to disciplined inquiry that nonetheless preserves an openness to discovery, creativity, and possibilities. What Schön (1978) terms "reflection-in-action," Friedman characterizes, somewhat more loosely, as a Piagetian process of assimilation and accommodation (p. 555). Countering an assumption that psychotherapists can adequately describe their work a priori and in generalized terms, Friedman (1988) identifies theories as tools, calling them "practical aids to attention, not abstract definitions" (p. 508). More specifically, he notes that a clinician best uses theory as a repertoire of "live metaphors, open-ended models, and imaginative maps" through which his unique and ambiguous relationship to this particular patient "is understood through the understanding of another thing" (p. 513). Such an understanding allows the therapist to impose some determinateness on an indeterminate situation without shutting off exploration of the particularities so essential to the enterprise.

Optimally, therapists use theory as a tool for listening and responding flexibly to their patients. At the same time that it serves to clarify the meaning of the interaction, though, Friedman posits that theory also contributes to ambiguity, by disrupting ordinary social expectations and thus sharply heightening therapists' and patients' awareness of what they do not know about themselves and each other. This gap between normal, expectable exchanges and the therapist's theoretically informed aloofness and opacity makes both participants more alert to what they want and expect.

Friedman's painstaking analyses of how therapists use theory to *both* foster and thwart comprehensible interactions takes him beyond Schön's characterization of reflection-in-action, to a more sophisticated comprehension of what Schön calls "back talk." For Friedman, patients respond not only to the specific interpretations and interventions their therapists make but also to their own more inchoate but irresistible striving for their therapists to satisfy their wishes. Psychotherapists use theory to withstand this pressure, to avoid responding "normally" to what their patients evoke. As a consequence, the therapist becomes for the patient an elusive interlocutor who both encourages and frustrates his deepest desires. For therapists, the constant effort to circumvent straightforward enactments of what patients long for helps them hear more clearly the specific motivations and meanings that inform patient-therapist interactions.

However, therapists cannot sustain ambiguity—or a commitment to "reflection-in-action"—by simply recognizing its value, even on persuasive theoretical grounds. They constantly juggle their own needs—for control, knowledge, and recognition—with a commitment to listening and responding to their patients' "back talk." Thus, no matter how experienced and confident a therapist feels about his practicing, he cannot avoid a sense of unease.[3] As Friedman (1988) put it:

---

[3] Friedman's recognition of the therapist's discomfort defends him against any charge that he is simply dressing up the blank screen in more contemporary clothes. A superficial similarity exists, though. In the traditional (one might say, stereotypical) view of psychoanalysis, the analyst makes no significant contribution to the patient's experience but, rather, serves as a foil for the patient's intrapsychic fantasies. Friedman also commits himself as a clinician to a relatively distant and opaque stance, as a means of disrupting and then identifying the patient's characteristic ways of relating. Unlike a blank screen, though, Friedman's analyst accepts as a given his involvement with his patient and makes no assumption that one can isolate intrapsychic phenomena. He defines psychotherapy as a distinctly abnormal *relationship* in which the therapist must constantly strive to remain sufficiently aloof. Far from being an end in itself, Friedman posits that the therapist's "mysteriousness" calls forth and makes available for inquiry the patient's wishes and desires.

> Most therapists know that one of the strongest forces in the consulting room, and the least controllable, is their own reluctance to give up a plausible understanding and agree to be lost all over again [p. 434]. . . . . Every time a therapist tries to correct an imbalance, he identifies with some stable image of a proper therapist. . . . . When in trouble, he will picture an unequivocal role [for himself] no matter how forcefully his theory insists that he remain ambiguous. The therapist needs to feel he is playing his part correctly, and that need is pressing and inescapable [p. 440].

In sum, the therapist's effort to withstand the pressures of his patient's demands has a double-edged significance. On one hand, it opens up a space in which he can imagine how his patient might change while, on the other, it seduces him into a variety of "disambiguating" postures that help him tolerate the radical open-endedness of his relationship with the patient.

Given that therapists neither can—nor should—deny their need for understanding and effectiveness, Friedman (1988) proposes that they develop other sources of satisfaction in their work, such as "an appetite for personal discovery and a delight in surprise" (p. 435). Such diversity of interest militates against the therapist's tendency to closure in his attitude toward his patient and his closely related concern that he act like a therapist.

Friedman develops most fully the importance of a therapist's multiple appetites in his consideration of psychotherapeutic training. Unlike Schön, Friedman is not primarily concerned with professional education, but he does conclude his project with thoughts about how to impart knowledge of the contradictory requirements of psychotherapeutic practicing. Whereas Schön emphasizes that therapists' expertise lies in their ability to define rather than solve problems, Friedman (without disagreeing) stresses the unanticipated difficulties and discoveries particular constructions of a problem might yield.

Friedman frames psychotherapeutic education in terms of a maxim and a dilemma. Given that no amount of study can clear up the essentially puzzling nature of psychoanalytic psychotherapy, he comments that "it is appropriately taught as a research project inquiring into its own nature." He continues, however, that "the trouble with this maxim is that therapy is difficult and upsetting, and trainees cannot be expected to begin it armed only with puzzles" (p. 539). Echoing Schön's (1983) instruction to "begin with a discipline, no matter how arbitrary" (p. 85), Friedman (1988) acknowledges the student's "need to begin with an unequivocal role" but, optimally with at least a preliminary appreciation that no one theory is the right one (p. 441). Correlatively, the supervisor's task is not to point out errors but to encourage flexibility by helping the trainee to articulate his several implicit beliefs about therapists, patients, and treatment. By examining a variety of theories as they surface in practicing, the student gains greater awareness of how theory shapes therapeutic goals and interventions and greater freedom in choosing "what trouble he prefers to what other trouble" (p. 442).

Far from an academic exercise, the power of clinical theory comes alive as students become increasingly aware of how they use it to regain their footing within the therapeutic situation. As my own case attests, actual interactions with patients constantly disturb the novice psychotherapist's beliefs about what he or she should do. Friedman challenges my claim, however, that I sometimes simply reacted without thinking. Persuaded that therapists always operate in terms of some theory or other, he sets out to alert supervisors to the need to make hidden assumptions available.

Committing oneself to one point of view necessarily precludes others, inviting the possibility of getting stuck or caught unawares. Friedman (1988) contends that the teacher of psychotherapy, like the practitioner, concerns himself with "spotting predicaments (for trainee and patient) and in seeing those problems in many alternative ways" (p. 551). This includes helping the student recognize and acknowledge that what he wants *from* his patient (given his theory) troubles their interactions as much as the difficulties the patient brings to the relationship. Through his own example, in discussing his own and his students' case material, the supervisor strives to foster a tolerance for the abnormality of the therapy relationship and an enthusiasm for self-discovery and surprise (Friedman, 1988, p. 546).

Theories of human potential, psychopathology, and therapeutic action more and less powerfully enable the therapist to interact meaningfully with his patient. Indeed, more than half of Friedman's book consists of his analyses of competing theories of mind, evaluated both as means for encouraging therapeutic direction and promise and as temporary resting spaces within this relentlessly puzzling business. More specifically, and consistent with his celebration of psychotherapeutic trouble, Friedman values more highly

those concepts—like resistance and certain versions of transference—that mitigate "the natural tendency of theory to smooth over
the dislocations of practice" by pushing therapists "to view the
tension more searchingly, and . . . [identify] how theory soothes it"
(p. 13). Thus, training must include not only a serious study of how
theory shapes and clashes with particular therapeutic encounters
but evaluative criteria by which the student can determine which
theories help more and which less.

Friedman's integration of the Piagetian notions of assimilation
and accommodation with psychoanalytic insight into how needs and
desires inform what and how we know, complements and deepens
Schön's "reflection-in-action" and suggests subtle variations on the
case study I have written. For example, Friedman's perspective aptly
frames an evaluative comparison of Masterson's theory with a milieu
approach in the specific terms of how I used each.

In explicating my use of Masterson's recommendations for the
inpatient treatment of borderline adolescents, I credited his theory
for providing a gambit in my conversation with a very confusing
patient and for affording me a sense of my function as her psychotherapist. At the same time, however, I described myself as responsive to "back talk" from Kay and the hospital staff, which made me
increasingly aware of serious limitations to Masterson's views. Specifically, I criticized the sameness of his case vignettes, his splitting
of the patient and therapist into all-bad and all-good, respectively,
and his authoritarian prescriptiveness about how the therapist
should act. Ultimately, I criticized myself for using Masterson's ideas
like blinders, to shut out feelings and perceptions that made me
uncomfortable.

Both Friedman and Schön provide frameworks within which I can
identify Masterson's theory as part of a repertoire of examples,
models, and clinical hypotheses that helped me to see a unique
situation as something familiar. Similarly, both theorists encourage
tolerant acceptance of my need, as a novice, to begin with a
discipline and a well-defined role. While Schön emphasizes the
encounter—or "conversation"—of ideas with particular circumstances, Friedman lingers on what we can learn when communication breaks down, when the patient's and therapist's purposes are
clearly at odds.

According to Friedman, my clinging to Masterson's prescription
for acting like a therapist does not indict me of self-deception in any

straightforward sense. Rather, Masterson's point of view reassured me that *as a therapist* I could understand and help Kay without getting stuck in the pathological relationships her behavior evoked. Only by becoming aware of and thwarting how I would respond to her if I were not her therapist could I withstand her demands and imagine as yet unrealized goals and directions for our work together.

From Friedman's perspective, I can accept with greater equanimity my reliance on Masterson's stereotypical case histories. Not only did they provide templates for my interpretations of Kay, but they motivated me to persevere in my efforts to achieve greater confidence in my intellectual mastery and practical efficacy (see Friedman, 1988, pp. 430-431). Even so, I stand by my conclusion that the milieu literature helped me more and think that here too Friedman furthers my ability to justify my allegiance.

Simply stated, the concepts of the split social field and parallel process offered me a vocabulary for interpersonal difficulties I found lacking in Masterson. Despite his descriptions of the borderline adolescent's rage and depression, Masterson portrayed the experienced therapist as calmly in charge, utterly certain of what he must do. In his view, therapeutic tension remained an essentially intrapsychic event, the result of unintegrated representations of a person's good and bad qualities; the patient projects his split images onto actual people he encounters, but the reality of these interactions does not contribute significantly to his experience.

By contrast, the concept of a multidirectional network allowed me to locate the tensions I felt in my therapeutic relationship with Kay within the context of the unit, the hospital, and my supervisors, among others. As discussed in detail in the previous chapter, because the milieu literature grew out of the interpersonalist tradition, it takes as central the mutual influence of therapists and patients. For me, the greater power of a psychotherapeutic milieu theory rested with how I could use its ideas both to comprehend and distance myself from the complexity of my reactions. By encouraging me to articulate my uses of these differing theories, Friedman enhanced the relative adaptability they afforded me in making sense of my work.

Friedman is careful to point out that he does not advocate teaching a piecemeal use of theory, nor does he believe that any theory that works in the moment is as good as any other. Consistent with his advocacy of models, metaphors, and imaginative maps, he discourages a grab bag approach to ideas that are isolated from theory. Without a context, a dynamic understanding of how various ideas relate to and influence each other, ideas can serve only as static images, not ways of envisioning a therapeutic situation with its horizon of possibilities.

Relatedly, Friedman (1988) deals skeptically with what he calls "phenomenologically concrete" theories that aim to represent psychotherapy as it actually unfolds. Much as he argues against the assumption that psychotherapy resembles "ordinary reality," he challenges the clinical utility of conceptualizations that come close to capturing the experience of therapeutic interactions (p. 437). For Friedman, as we have seen, the therapist must sustain the tension between his ideas and his experience if he hopes to preserve the therapeutic space in which the treatment unfolds. The therapist relies on theory in order to imagine his patient's potentialities, not just to describe what is actually the case.

Friedman's warning about these possible misuses of theory suggests that he would judge my use of projective identification quite harshly. First of all, I most certainly did not locate this notion within a more comprehensive system, whether Klein's, Ogden's, or one of my supervisor's. I did consider its implications for my views on myself and my patient but not in a way that was well thought out or coherent. Second, and perhaps more damning from Friedman's perspective, for a time I understood projective identification as a literal description of my relationship with Kay; indeed, I almost believed that it existed in the very air we breathed.

I agree with Friedman's implicit assessment of my use of projective identification up to a point. During an especially stressful period of my training, I clung to the notion that I "contained" Kay's disowned affects and that my task was to metabolize and feed them back to her. To the extent that I concretely equated what I then felt with what Kay was putting into me, I let myself be seduced into believing that I appeared as the theory described. More seriously, I risked responding too literally to Kay's demands, thereby losing a distance and ambiguity essential to our work. As a result, I shut out other valuable perspectives—including hers—on what was going on between us and in the milieu.

Even so, I cannot ignore the positive benefits that accrued to my use of projective identification. At the time that projective identification seemed magically to save me, I badly needed to identify "with some stable image of a proper therapist" (Friedman, 1988, p. 440) in order to persist in what had become a far too painful pursuit. To criticize this notion as too phenomenological at the level of theory discounts the constructive use to which I put it in actually tolerating the ambiguities of my situation. Similarly, to criticize my use of projective identification as providing too static a view of my patient's possibilities for change minimizes the central role it played as I explored the potentialities of my role as a psychotherapist.

More generally, I contend that Friedman's insistence that therapists use complete theories and not isolated ideas detracts from his appreciation of "reflection-in-action." I think he fails to make a crucial distinction between phenomenologically concrete notions and good phenomenological *descriptions* of how theory shapes and responds to the particularities of what psychotherapists do. Finally, I am convinced that a phenomenological case study of both therapists' and patients' linked efforts at assimilation and accommodation would contribute to the training goals to which Friedman feels committed.

Ironically, in accusing Friedman of not differentiating a phenomenologically concrete theory from a case study that depicts theorizing-in-action, I am faulting him for not following through on the promise of his book's introductory remarks. He knows better than I that psychotherapists write least about what they know best (1988, p. 5), seldom conveying the constant tensions of working with patients. While Friedman brilliantly explains why *theory* cannot and should not accomplish this aim, he ultimately does not explore alternative rhetorics that psychotherapists can draw upon to write. A case study can acknowledge the autonomy and integrity of theories while simultaneously demonstrating how therapists put them to work.

LAST WORD

When I last saw Kay, she was dressed all in white and laughing. She had cut her blond, wavy hair very short, and no makeup covered the pale freckles that the summer sun had beckoned. We had formally "said good-byes" in our last session the day before, hamming it up playing a duet of "Heart and Soul" on the unit's piano and stepping back from the momentousness of this long-prepared-for separation. Officially finished with my training, I had returned to State for one final planning meeting with the team and CAS. I was glad for one last glimpse of the young woman with whom I had learned so much.

Kay was getting on the elevator and was on her way to the gynecologist's to have cryosurgery (the use of liquid nitrogen to destroy her abnormal cervical cells by freezing). She was doped up on tranquilizers in anticipation of the discomfort. As she playfully tried to push all the elevator buttons, she swayed groggily against the milieu worker who accompanied her. The worker, spying me, remarked gruffly but not unkindly, on my apparent inability to get myself gone. I said something—"hello," "good-bye"—I cannot remember what. Kay continued to giggle as the elevator doors shut.

As far as I know, the cryosurgery was successful. Kay was released from A-2 about six weeks later to a residential placement in a western state that sounded as well suited to her needs as we could realistically hope for. Organized to promote its residents' increasing autonomy, it also had a restricted unit where they could stay when their self-control was endangered. One staff member remarked, as she reviewed the brochures, that the place looked more like a resort than a placement for disturbed adolescents. While I doubted that it would be so luxurious or pleasurable, I had some assurance that it would be at least as safe and helpful as what we had been able to offer.

I have not heard from Kay directly since our encounter at the elevator. She called the unit several times, though, after she left. As the nurse supervisor remarked when I spoke with her last, Kay seems to have done as well as we could expect.

REFERENCES

Bettelheim, B. (1974), *Home for the Heart*. New York: Knopf.
_____ (1975), *The Uses of Enchantment*. New York: Vintage.
Bion, W. R. (1959), *Experiences in Groups*. London: Tavistock.
_____ (1967), *Second Thoughts*. New York: Aronson.
Casement, P. (1985), *On Learning from the Patient*. London: Tavistock.
Coser, R. L. (1979), *Training in Ambiguity: Learning Through Doing in a Mental Hospital*. New York: Free Press.
Erikson, E. H. (1956), The problem of ego identity. In: *Essential Papers on Borderline Disorders*, ed. M. Stone. New York: New York University Press, 1986, pp. 229–242.
_____ (1964), *Insight and Responsibility*. New York: Norton.
Friedman, L. (1978), Trends in the psychoanalytic theory of treatment. *Psychoanal. Quart.*, 47:524–567.
_____ (1982), The interplay of evocation. Presented to the Postgraduate Center for Mental Health, Cornell Medical School, New York City.
_____ (1988), *The Anatomy of Psychotherapy*. Hillsdale, NJ: The Analytic Press.
Gediman, H. & Wolkenfeld, F. (1980), The parallelism phenomenon in psychoanalysis and supervision.*Psychoanal. Quart.*, 49:234–255.
Gill, M. M. (1983), The interpersonal paradigm and the degree of the therapist's involvement. *Contemp. Psychoanal.*, 19:200–237.
_____ (1985), The interactional aspect of transference: Range of application. In: *The Transference in Psychotherapy: Clinical Management*, ed. E. A. Schwaber. New York: International Universities Press, pp. 87–102.
_____ & Hoffman, I. Z. (1982), *Analysis of Transference II*. New York: International Universities Press.
Greenberg, J. & Mitchell, S. (1983), *Object Relations in Psychoanalytic Theory*. Cambridge, MA: Harvard University Press.
Grey, A. & Fiscalini, J. (1987), Parallel process as transference-countertransference interaction. *Psychoanal. Psychol.*, 4:131–144.
Hoffman, I. Z. (1983), The patient as interpreter of the analyst's experience. *Contemp. Psychoanal.*, 19:389–422.

_____ (1990), In the eye of the beholder. *Contemp. Psychoanal.*, 26:291–304.

_____ (1991), Discussion: Toward a social-constructivist view of the psychoanalytic situation. *Psychoanal. Dial.*, 1:74–105.

Keith, C. R. (1968), The therapeutic alliance in child psychotherapy. *J. Amer. Acad. Child Psychiat.*, 7:31–43.

Kernberg, O. F. (1978a), The diagnosis of borderline conditions in adolescence. In: *Adolescent Psychiatry, Vol. 6*, ed. J. Feinstein & P. Giovacchini. Chicago: University of Chicago Press, pp. 298–319.

_____ (1978b), Leadership and organizational functioning: Organizational regression. *Internat. J. Group Psychother.*, 28:3—25.

Kierkegaard, S. (1944), *Either/Or*, trans. D. F. Swenson. Princeton, NJ: Princeton University Press.

Klein, M. (1946), Notes on some schizoid mechanisms. *Internat. J. Psycho-Anal.*, 27:99–110.

_____ (1955), On identification. In: *Envy and Gratitude and Other Works, 1946–1963*. New York: Delacorte, 1975, pp. 141–175.

Klein, R. H. (1981), The patient-staff community meeting: A tea-party with the Mad Hatter. *Internat. J. Group Psychother.*, 31:205–222.

Kobler, A. L. & Stotland, E. (1964), *The End of Hope*. New York: Free Press.

Kohut, H. (1979), The two analyses of Mr. Z. *Internat. J. Psycho-Anal.*, 60:3–27.

Kulish, N. M. (1985–1986), Projective identification: A concept overburdened. *Internat. J. Psychoanal. Psychother.*, 11:79–104.

Lerner, S. (1979), The excessive need to treat: A countertherapeutic force in psychiatric hospital treatment. *Bull. Menn. Clin.*, 43:463–471.

Levenson, E. (1972), *The Fallacy of Understanding*. New York: Basic Books.

_____ (1981), Facts or fantasies: The nature of psychoanalytic data. *Contemp. Psychoanal.*, 17:486–500.

_____ (1982), Language and healing. In: *Curative Factors in Dynamic Psychotherapy*, ed. S. Slipp. New York: McGraw-Hill, pp. 91–103.

Mahler, M. S., Pine, F. & Bergman, A. (1975), *The Psychological Birth of the Human Infant*. New York: Basic Books.

Marohn, R. C., Dalle-Molle, D., McCarter, E. & Linn, D. (1980), *Juvenile Delinquents: Psychodynamic Assessment and Hospital Treatment*. New York: Brunner/Mazel.

Masterson, J. F. (1972), *Treatment of the Borderline Adolescent*. New York: Wiley-Interscience.

_____ (1975), The splitting mechanism of the borderline adolescent: Developmental and clinical aspects. In: *Borderline States in Psychiatry*, ed. J. E. Mack. New York: Grune & Stratton, pp. 93–101.

_____ (1980), *From Borderline Adolescent to Functioning Adult*. New York: Brunner/Mazel.

_____ (1983), *Countertransference and Psychotherapeutic Technique: Teaching Seminars on Psychotherapy of the Borderline Adult*. New York: Brunner/Mazel.

_____ & Rinsley, D. B. (1975), The role of the mother in the genesis and psychic structure of the borderline personality. *Internat. J. Psycho-Anal.*, 56:163–178.

McCaughan, D. L. (1985), Teaching and learning adolescent psychotherapy: Adolescent, therapist, and milieu. *Adoles. Psychiatry*, 12:414–433.

Merleau-Ponty, M. (1945), *Phénoménologie de la Perception*. Paris: Librarie Gallimard.

Mitchell, S. A. (1988), *Relational Concepts in Psychoanalysis*. New York: Basic Books.

Ogden, T. H. (1982), *Projective Identification and Psychotherapeutic Technique*. New York: Aronson.

Pine, F. (1974), On the concept "borderline" in children. *The Psychoanalytic Study of the Child*, 29:341–368. New Haven, CT: Yale University Press.

_____ (1983), Borderline syndromes in childhood: A working nosology and its therapeutic implications. In: *The Borderline Child*, ed. K. S. Robson. New York: McGraw-Hill, pp. 83–100.

Racker, H. (1968). *Transference and Countertransference*. New York: International Universities Press.

Rinsley, D. B. (1982), *Borderline and Other Self Disorders*. New York: Aronson.

Sachs, D. & Shapiro, S. (1974), Comments on teaching psychoanalytic psychotherapy in a residency training program. *Psychoanal. Quart.*, 43:51–76.

_____ (1976), On parallel processes in therapy and teaching. *Psychoanal. Quart.*, 45:394–415.

Sandler, J. (1976), Countertransference and role-responsiveness. *Internat. Rev. Psycho-Anal.*, 3:43–47.

Schön, D. A. (1983), *The Reflective Practitioner: How Professionals Think in Action*. New York: Basic Books.

_____ (1987), *Educating the Reflective Practitioner*. San Francisco, CA: Jossey-Bass.

Searles, H. (1979), *Countertransference and Related Subjects*. New York: International Universities Press.

_____ (1986), The countertransference with the borderline patient. In: *Essential Papers on Borderline Disorders*, ed. M. H. Stone. New York: New York University Press, pp. 498–526.

Segal, H. (1974), *Introduction to the Work of Melanie Klein*. New York: Basic Books.

Stanton, A. H. & Schwartz, M. S. (1954), *The Mental Hospital*. New York: Basic Books.

Stern, D. B. (1990), Courting surprise. *Contemp. Psychoanal.*, 26:452–478.

_____ (1991), A philosophy for the embedded analyst. *Contemp. Psychoanal.*, 27:51–80.

Stone, M. H., ed. (1986), *Essential Papers on Borderline Disorders*. New York: New York University Press.

Sugarman, A. & Lerner, H. D. (1980), Reflections on the current state of the borderline concept. In: *Borderline Phenomena and the Rorschach Test*, ed. J. Kwawer, H. Lerner, P. Lerner & A. Sugarman. New York: International Universities Press, pp. 11–37.

Sullivan, H. S. (1940), *Conceptions of Modern Psychiatry*. New York: Norton.

_____ (1953), *The Interpersonal Theory of Psychiatry*. New York: Norton.

_____ (1954), *The Psychiatric Interview*. New York: Norton.

Tansey, M. J. & Burke, W. F. (1989), *Understanding Countertransference*. Hillsdale, NJ: The Analytic Press.

Vela, R. M., Gottlieb, E. H. & Gottlieb, H. P. (1983), Borderline syndromes in childhood: A critical review. In: *The Borderline Child*, ed. K. S. Robson. New York: McGraw-Hill, pp. 31–48.

AFTERWORD

Glen O. Gabbard

Francis Bacon once noted that even wrong theories are better than chaos. The foregoing account of Rita McCleary's treatment of Kay is a saga involving a therapist's search for a theory that will lead her out of chaos. In her quest, she encounters a series of theoretical constructs, each of which is "wrong" in one way or another. Nevertheless, Dr. McCleary seems to glean something useful from each of her forays into theory and creates order out of the chaos surrounding her.

In counterpoint to the therapist-in-search-of-a-theory theme, a subtext emerges as the plot unfolds. This subtext is essentially a story of how the needs of patients, trainees, and staff members converge and collide in the crucible of long-term psychoanalytically oriented hospital treatment. Thanks to Dr. McCleary's courage and forthrightness in revealing her own internal experience as she sought to make sense of her environment, the reader gains a glimpse of the neophyte therapist's struggle to develop a sense of professional self-confidence in the face of enormous adversity.

In this brief attempt to put Dr. McCleary's experience into some larger context, I will touch on both the major theme concerning the role of theory in practice and the subtextual theme involving the human dimension of conflicting needs in the hospital setting.

Glen O. Gabbard, M.D. is Director, C. F. Menninger Hospital, and Training and Supervising Analyst, Topeka Institute for Psychoanalysis.

CHAOS, BORDERLINE PERSONALITY DISORDER,
AND THEORY

Few diagnostic entities have spawned as much theorizing as has the borderline personality disorder. Its protean nature is undoubtedly responsible to some extent for the reams of paper devoted to psychodynamic explanations, but the diversity of formulations brought to bear on a particular disorder is often directly proportional to the degree of chaos it engenders. Borderline patients veritably overwhelm their treaters. They evoke a feeling in therapists and hospital staff that their suffering could be alleviated if only the treater would say or do exactly the right thing. Because borderline patients spend much of their time in a paranoid-schizoid mode, in which there is no sense of self-continuity, they engender a sense of urgency—everything must be done now! The punishment inflicted on therapists who do not respond to those immediate needs is an affect storm that may induce in those treaters intense feelings of guilt and responsibility. Moreover, the twin fears of merger and object loss cause borderline patients to oscillate between closeness and distance in a manner that is highly confusing to others, who are deeply perplexed by the patients' rapidly changing "selves." Finally, borderline patients deal with their own inability to tolerate strong affective experience by inducing corresponding emotional states— some would say "illnesses"—in their treaters.

It was just such a clinical picture that led Dr. McCleary to grasp for a life raft of theory to avoid drowning in a sea of uncertainty. Her choice of Masterson's formulation is understandable. She discovered a master clinician who appeared to have all the answers. A specific developmental lesion could be identified. The maternal tendency to reward clinging and to withdraw from efforts at autonomy leads to a specific intrapsychic constellation of part-object-relations units. This internal object world is then systematically examined through predictable stages in the psychotherapy manifested by specific transferences.

Unfortunately, Dr. McCleary's appropriation of Masterson's theory quickly became problematic because the formulation does not fit the clinical data. To treat borderline patients effectively, therapists must be willing to tolerate long periods of ambiguity. Bollas (1987) characterized this therapeutic posture as follows:

> We must acknowledge more frankly that in the midst of countertransference experiencing the analyst may for a very long time indeed exist in an unknowable region. To be sure, he may know that he is being cumulatively coerced by the patient's transference towards some interpersonal environment, but analyses rarely proceed with such clarity that the clinician knows in *statu nascendi* what and whom he is meant to become [p. 200].

Beginning therapists too often feel compelled to choose a theoretical model prematurely in their effort to make order out of the transference-countertransference chaos. They may not take the necessary time to study carefully the relationship between the patient's history and the current difficulties.

Kay's actual childhood experiences, for example, bore little or no relationship to the model postulated by Masterson. Masterson's theory requires an overinvolved mother who provides nurturance and emotional support until the rapprochement subphase of separation-individuation occurs at around 18 months of age. At this point, the mother is threatened by the autonomy of the child's potential and withdraws her love and support. By contrast, Kay's childhood was characterized not by overinvolvement, but by gross neglect and abuse.

An examination of Kay's childhood reveals another frequent problem in the application of theory to technique in the treatment of borderline patients. As with most cases of borderline personality disorder, no phase-specific problem in parenting can be documented. Gunderson (1984) observed that a global parental failure in all developmental phases generally occurs in the families of patients with borderline pathology. Indeed, even Mahler herself (Mahler and Kaplan, 1977) eschewed a reductionistic conceptualization of the etiology and pathogenesis of borderline personality disorder as stemming from difficulties in one developmental phase.

Kay's situation reflects yet another problematic trend in the psychoanalytic literature on borderline personality disorder. Too often the psychodynamic theorizing is completely disconnected from the data accrued from empirical investigations. Kay fits a common profile in contemporary practice that has been bolstered by the findings of five different studies. Westen et al. (1990) studied records of inpatient adolescents diagnosed with borderline person-

ality disorder and discovered that over 50% had evidence of physical abuse, sexual abuse, or both as children. Similarly, Herman,
Perry, and van der Kolk (1989) found that 68% of a sample of 21
borderline patients had been sexually abused as children, 71% had
been physically abused, and 62% had witnessed serious domestic
violence.

Early separation from caretakers has also been implicated in
borderline psychopathology. Zanarini et al. (1989) found that 74%
of the patients with borderline personality disorder in their sample
had experienced loss or prolonged separation from a caretaker
before the age of 18. Their investigation also revealed a high level of
verbal, physical, and sexual abuse in childhood, as did another study
by Ogata et al. (1990). Emotional neglect is a common feature in
these studies, typified by the findings of Zweig-Frank and Paris
(1991) demonstrating that borderline patients are significantly more
likely than a control group to remember their parents as having been
uncaring.

If we examine the empirical research as a whole, we reach the
unmistakable conclusion that several pathways lead to the development of borderline personality disorder. Some combination of neglect, early separation, physical abuse, verbal abuse, and sexual
abuse is often involved, and usually these factors apply throughout
development rather than in one phase only. To be fair to Masterson,
the work of Zweig-Frank and Paris suggests that some patients
experienced overcontrol in childhood that may have led them to be
anxious about abandonment. The overcontrol, however, generally
involved both parents rather than only the mother.

This discussion of research data is not idle, ivory-tower discourse.
The risk of imposing one's preferred theory on the patient is that the
patient will experience *depersonification,* a term applied to borderline adolescents by Rinsley (1980), Masterson's erstwhile collabora-
tor. Children who are depersonified are treated by their parents as
though they were someone other than who they are. Rinsley identified this pattern of parenting in the backgrounds of borderline
adolescents. Hence, the glib use of a superimposed theory may
retraumatize these patients, many of whom grew up in households
where their inner world was a container for parental projections.

It is to Dr. McCleary's credit that she discovered the poor fit
between her patient's psychological world and Masterson's theory.
She allowed herself to be "supervised" by her patient. The sensitive

therapist must always listen to the patient's "talking back" to make midcourse correction. We must never lose track of Freud's dictum that in some way the patient is always right.

EXTERNALIZATION OF THE INTERNAL WORLD

One of the great values of intensive hospital treatment is that the drama of the patient's internal object world is played out on the stage of the milieu. The borderline patient's chief defense mechanisms, splitting and projective identification, are instrumental to this process (Gabbard, 1986, 1988, 1989, 1992a). Split-off self- and object representations are projectively disavowed and "deposited" into various staff members through the process of projective identification. Staff members working in the milieu typically feel "bullied" or coerced into assuming a particular role vis-à-vis the patient. In this manner, the patient's childhood experiences—or, to be more precise, the internalized version of those experiences—are recapitulated in the interpersonal relationships that develop with staff members.

The "noise" created by Kay in the milieu beautifully illustrates this process. As Dr. McCleary observes, Kay's hospitalization was characterized by a series of "leavings." Because of the recurrent trauma she had experienced during her childhood, with one parental departure after another, Kay internalized an object relationship involving an abandoning object and an abandoned self. By constantly eloping from the unit, she re-created this internal object world, with one significant difference: This time *she* was the one doing the leaving; Dr. McCleary was the one left behind. In other words, Kay assumed the role of the abandoning object, while her therapist was coerced into being the abandoned self. Similarly, Kay's experiences of abuse in childhood were transformed into contemporary versions in which she tormented her therapist and the hospital staff so they would suffer as she had.

This pattern of projective identification is a form of active mastery over passively experienced trauma and is one of the major motivational forces behind the recapitulation of internal object relations in the hospital milieu. Kay's behavior, however, also illustrates another unconscious motivation—a cry for help. Projective identification is not simply a defense mechanism. It is also a forerunner of empathy and therefore a means of communication. Kay was letting Dr. McCleary know what being Kay felt like and was indirectly asking for help. Finally, an implicit wish for transformation also occurs in the repetition of internal object relations: Maybe this time will be different, and the longed-for parents will emerge in the treatment relationships. Old objects will be changed into new objects.

Dr. McCleary rapidly discovered what all psychotherapists soon learn in the long-term intensive hospital treatment of borderline patients. We find the patient by looking within ourselves (Bollas, 1987, 1989). Although analysts working exclusively with neurotic outpatients find the concept of projective identification difficult to grasp, therapists of highly disturbed inpatients typically find it to be an accurate formulation of their own experience. Dr. McCleary also came to recognize that containing and metabolizing the patient's projections may have powerful therapeutic effects even when interpretation is not involved. During the chair-slamming session, Dr. McCleary demonstrated to Kay that she (Dr. McCleary) could manage the intense feelings that Kay could not handle. Projective identification often emerges as an effort by the patient to destroy links between the affect and the patient because the feelings are unbearable. When patients observe their therapists' capacity to bear those same feelings, linkage may be restored as the patients "re-own" their feelings (Carpy, 1989; Gabbard, 1991). This process occurs daily when milieu staff make a concerted effort to process what is going on with the patient rather than to respond in a "knee-jerk" manner.

In her discussion of projective identification, Dr. McCleary refers to it as a concept that isolated her from the other staff; she regards it as essentially a process occurring in dyads. Yet, there is a literature that applies projective identification to groups (Horwitz, 1983), to families (Shapiro et al., 1975; Zinner and Shapiro, 1972, 1974; Slipp, 1984, 1988), and to the treatment staff of institutions (Gabbard, 1989, 1992a). Scapegoating is a common manifestation of projective identification in groups and on hospital units. For example, Kay was a convenient repository for the staff members' own unacceptable and disavowed impulses—by controlling the unit's scapegoat, they could maintain an unconscious illusion of control over their own distasteful aspects. Patients serve as containers for staff projections as well as vice-versa.

The key to managing splitting in the milieu is the recognition of

multiple projective identification processes (Gabbard, 1989). Because certain staff members viewed Kay as "bad" (i.e., sociopathic)
and others viewed her as "sick" (i.e., borderline), a specific self-
representation in Kay may have coercively elicited a particular
corresponding object representation in some staff members who
viewed her as sociopathic, while a separate self-representation elicited a different corresponding object response in others. Each staff
member has a different piece of the puzzle, and only through an
integrated effort involving frank sharing in staff meetings about
different views of the patient can the splitting processes be examined and understood. The absence of regularly scheduled process
meetings for all staff members severely hampered the integration of
the disparate aspects of Kay in her hospital treatment. A strong,
psychoanalytically informed unit leader needs to set a tone of open
discussion involving the sharing of intense emotional reactions and
the positive labeling of those reactions as important diagnostic
information (Gabbard, 1989). When staff members are educated
about splitting and projective identification, a messy, confusing
situation suddenly becomes entirely understandable.

The true test of a theory lies in its usefulness. Theories do not
exist in a realm of absolute truth. They are valid only if they make
clinical situations understandable and their premises are internally
consistent with the available data. By this standard, the theoretical
construct of projective identification is an extraordinarily valuable
tool in hospital treatment. Nevertheless, we must heed Dr. Mc-
Cleary's cautionary note regarding the limitations of theory and
recognize that some clinical interactions in the milieu will not
readily lend themselves to this framework.

THE INTRAPSYCHIC VERSUS THE INTERPERSONAL

As Dr. McCleary aptly points out, the classic Stanton and Schwartz
study (1954) continues to be highly relevant to contemporary inpatient treatment. These two investigators demonstrated persuasively
that covert staff disagreement can result in acting-out behavior by
the patient. The difficulty with their formulation, however, is that
just as psychoanalytic clinicians before them had neglected the
social forces, Stanton and Schwartz failed to incorporate the intrapsychic elements inherent in the split social field. The concept of
projective identification provides a bridge between the intrapsychic

and the interpersonal (Ogden, 1982). In other words, the social forces described by Stanton and Schwartz can also be understood as the externalization of intrapsychic tensions through projective iden-tification. In a situation of covert staff disagreement, staff members involved in the conflict commonly keep their anger at each other under tight control. A patient who is the subject of disagreement may then erupt in an explosion of rage as the result of unconscious coercion by the parties in conflict. Their own anger is thereby projectively disavowed and acted out by the patient.

Dr. McCleary suggests, "It seemed increasingly plausible, in-stead, that the controversies that surrounded her hospitalization were the *source* and not the *result* of her agitation and flight. Our dissension had less to do with her *intrapsychic* instability, in other words, than with the instabilities inherent in the *interpersonal* situa-tion in which we placed her." This view postulates an "either/or" relationship between the intrapsychic and interpersonal that, I be-lieve, is unwarranted. When splitting and projective identification occur in the milieu, the targets of the projections are not randomly identified. Patients typically project certain aspects of themselves onto a staff member who represents a "good fit" with the projection (Gabbard, 1989). Borderline patients in particular have a kind of "radar" that enables them to detect which staff members tend to be more punitive as well as those who are more permissive. The former are likely targets for "bad object" projections, while the latter may be assigned "good object" projections. Similarly, preexisting staff disagreement, based on philosophical or personality differences, provides a fertile field for any patient admitted to a unit who is unconsciously looking for suitable objects in the environment (Gabbard, 1989).

In regard to Hoffman's (1983) concern that the classical notion of the blank screen has been supplanted by the concept of the empty container, I would agree that an "empty container" is no more viable than a "blank screen." No mystical transfer of mental con-tents occurs in projective identification. Even when therapists feel coerced into responses that seem distinctly ego alien, their coerced responses do not literally come from the patient. Rather, disavowed or repressed aspects of themselves are activated by certain forms of interpersonal pressure by the patient. We all harbor an internal cast of characters that includes murderers and abusers as well as saints and rescuers. Borderline patients are expert at summoning these ghosts within us to play a role in the patients' internal drama.

THE CONFLUENCE OF CONFLICTING NEEDS

The needs of inexperienced therapists frequently are in conflict with those of the veteran unit staff, who provide a sense of history and continuity to the inpatient milieu. Issues emerging from this clash include the following: Who is in charge of the patient's treatment? How are decisions made regarding the patient's management? Whose interventions are most crucial to the ultimate outcome of treatment? Who truly understands the patient's needs? The last issue is emblematic of a serious risk in intensive psychiatric hospital treatment, namely, that the patient's needs may be lost in a skirmish between staff members. What is poignantly apparent in Dr. Mc-Cleary's compelling account is that a host of narcissistic vulnerabilities—in patients, staff, and trainees—are laid bare in the day-to-day task of treating the "untreatable" patient.

A psychiatric hospital setting is often compared to a family. Within this metaphor, a commonality between the family and the hospital is that one's own needs are competing with a host of others. Although treaters may attempt to convince themselves that they are suppressing their own needs in the interest of serving the patient's needs, rarely is that situation realizable in the treatment of borderline patients. Staff members often have the sense that they are desperately trying to survive in an emotionally charged atmosphere of contempt, rage, hate, pain, longing, and grief.

To make matters more complex, new therapists arrive on the scene with a set of unconscious needs that are intrinsic to their choice of a career as a psychotherapist. Dr. McCleary was sufficiently in touch with her own needs to sense that she was highly invested in being a rescuer of a patient whom she needed to see as "innocent," a victim of the abuse of others. She also became aware of her need to be seen as "nice" and to like her patient. Much to her therapist's chagrin, Kay preferred to see her as an oppressive, evil witch. In response, Dr. McCleary attempted to become even more caring and considerate.

Psychotherapists are often drawn to the field because the practice of psychotherapy provides a convenient defense against sadism, hatred, and aggression (Schafer, 1954; Menninger, 1957; McLaugh-lin, 1961; Gabbard, 1991). The role of the idealized, omnipotent rescuer, however, places a great burden on the patient to be the carrier of all hate in the dyad. To be truly helpful to the patient, the therapist needs to embrace a position that is intermediate between the old object and the new object (Greenberg, 1986). Only if the therapist is partly experienced as an imperfect object from the past will the patient have the opportunity to work through the conflictual issues in the transference (Casement, 1990; Gabbard, 1990, 1992a).

Dr. McCleary soon learned that it was not tenable for her to assume the role of the healthy member of the dyad while the patient took the sick role. She found that she had much in common with the patient and even identified similar struggles in herself, such as her own wish to flee as the patient had. In this discovery, Dr. McCleary identified one of the key principles of psychoanalytically informed hospital treatment, namely, that we are more like the patient than different. Searles (1986) made the following observation:

> It is essential that the analyst acknowledge to himself that even the patient's most severe psychopathology has some counterpart, per-haps relatively small by comparison but by no means insignificant, in his own *real* personality functioning. We cannot help the borderline patient, for example, to become well if we are trying unwittingly to use him as a receptacle for our own most deeply unwanted personality components, and trying essentially to require him to bear the burden of all the severe psychopathology, in the whole relationship [p. 22].

The new therapist's need to master sadism and aggression is only one of a myriad of needs that are activated in the hospital setting. Professional self-esteem is on the line when one enters a new inpatient unit. In the treatment of borderline patients, one often faces a quandary: Should one's principal alliance be with the staff in the service of presenting a "united front," or should it be with the patient, even if that places one at odds with the staff? The staff members in the hospital often have a different agenda than the trainees. Staff members are more or less permanent fixtures in the milieu; trainees are to be "endured." Yet, despite this defensive posture, attachment to the trainees occurs, and they are faced with repeated losses at the end of each academic year. Just as therapists long to establish order from chaos by the use of theory, hospital staff hope to establish order through "structure." Rules and procedures must be followed. Rule Number 1 is that decisions must be made by the "team," an admonition to trainees that they had better not function independently.

In the face of repeated devaluation and contempt from a unit full of borderline patients, the staff struggles to maintain a sense of self-esteem and value. The accusation of splitting that reduced Dr. McCleary to tears was at one level a communication to the novice therapist that the nursing staff felt they weren't being sufficiently valued by her. They feared that she was siding with the patient against them. Dr. McCleary wept because she felt that she, in turn, was not valued and appreciated by the nursing staff.

Throughout her year on the unit, Dr. McCleary jockeyed between a position of isolation and one of solidarity with the team. She describes the deleterious effects associated with either extreme. The optimal position is one of team membership but not solidarity at all cost. Therapists need to view themselves as a part of a group engaged in a common task, but also as members who can freely disagree without fear of repercussion. Therapists of borderline patients often hide behind a mask of confidentiality, but isolation from the team is a set-up for problems with splitting. A more sensible stance is at the middle ground, where discretion, rather than absolute confidentiality, is the by word. I have yet to see a patient who truly objects to this arrangement. It is generally more of a staff issue than a patient issue and pivots around the existence of mutual respect among members of the treatment team.

Therapists must also be mindful that the nursing staff have needs of their own that are entirely legitimate. Nurses regularly run the risk of assault, racial and ethnic slurs, out-of-control behavior that may injure other patients, and responsibility for suicide. The need to have an orderly milieu and firm structure at times may represent a countertransference posture, but it is also a means of preserving safety and predictability in a difficult environment. The more the therapist can empathize with unit staff and understand their needs, the less the possibility that splitting will disrupt the treatment.

CONCLUSION

One cannot read Dr. McCleary's moving account without reflecting on the contemporary crisis in psychiatric hospital treatment. It is increasingly difficult to find hospitals that are willing to undertake long-term psychoanalytically oriented treatment in the current climate of "quick fixes" and cost containment. In the public sector, state hospitals work toward rapid discharge and typically regard borderline patients as "not appropriate" for their treatment programs. In the private sector, insurance companies and managed-care firms limit hospitalization to "acute medical necessity" and continue to slash mental health benefits.

Despite these changes in the economic forces that drive mental health services, a significant subgroup of psychiatric patients— perhaps 10 to 30%—fail to respond to brief hospitalization and require extended inpatient treatment (Gabbard, 1992b). Many of these patients are, like Kay, seriously self-destructive borderline patients whose only hope is to find a holding environment. As Marcus (1987) eloquently stated, "The problem with the sickest patients is that the affects are uncontainable by a single individual" (p. 251). Only a group of reliable, sturdy staff members can handle the tasks of containment, holding, and processing of the affects generated by this segment of the patient population. It is a sad commentary that society does not value this service as much as an organ transplant or bypass surgery. Let us hope that Dr. McCleary's powerful account of Kay's treatment is read widely and carefully.

REFERENCES

Bollas, C. (1987), *The Shadow of the Object: Psychoanalysis of the Unthought Known*. New York: Columbia University Press.
_____ (1989), *Forces of Destiny: Psychoanalysis and Human Idiom*. Northvale, NJ: Aronson.
Carpy, D.V. (1989), Tolerating the countertransference: A mutative process. *Internat. Rev. Psycho-Anal.*, 70:287–294.
Casement, P.J. (1990), The meeting of needs in psychoanalysis. *Psychoanal. Inq.*, 10:325–346.
Gabbard, G.O. (1986), The treatment of the "special" patient in a psychoanalytic hospital. *Internat. Rev. Psycho-Anal.*, 13:333–347.
_____ (1988), A contemporary perspective on psychoanalytically informed hospital treatment. *Hosp. & Community Psychiat.*, 39:1291–1295.
_____ (1989), Splitting in hospital treatment. *Amer. J. Psychiat.*, 146:444–451.
_____ (1990), *Psychodynamic Psychiatry in Clinical Practice*. Washington, DC: American Psychiatric Press.
_____ (1991), Technical approaches to transference hate in the analysis of borderline patients. *Internat. J. Psycho-Anal.*, 72:625–638.

_____ (1992a), The therapeutic relationship in psychiatric hospital treatment. *Bull. Menn. Clin.*, 56:4–19.

_____ (1992b), Comparative indications for brief and extended hospitalization. *Review of Psychiatry Vol. 11*, ed. A. Tasman & M. Riba. Washington, DC: American Psychiatric Press, pp. 503–517.

Greenberg, J.R. (1986), Theoretical models and the analyst's neutrality. *Contemp. Psychoanal.*, 22:87–106.

Gunderson, J. (1984), *Borderline Personality Disorder*. Washington, DC: American Psychiatric Press.

Herman, J.L., Perry, J.C. & van der Kolk, B.A. (1989), Childhood trauma in borderline personality disorder. *Amer. J. Psychiat.*, 146:490–495.

Hoffman, I.Z. (1983), The patient as interpreter of the analyst's experience. *Contemp. Psychoanal.*, 19:389–422.

Horwitz, L. (1983), Projective identification in dyads and groups. *Internat. Group Psychother.*, 33:259–279.

Mahler, M.S. & Kaplan, L.J. (1977), Developmental aspects in the assessment of narcissistic and so-called borderline personalities. In: *Borderline Personality Disorders: The Concept, the Syndrome, the Patient*, ed. P.L. Hartocollis. New York: International Universities Press, pp. 71–85.

Marcus, E. (1987), Relationship of illness and intensive hospital treatment to length of stay. *Psychiat. Clin. North America*, 10:247–255.

McLaughlin, J.T. (1961), The analyst and the Hippocratic Oath. *J. Amer. Psychoanal. Assn.*, 9:106–123.

Menninger, K. (1957), Psychological factors in the choice of medicine as a profession. *Bull. Menn. Clin.*, 21:51–58.

Ogata, S.N., Silk, K.R., Goodrich, S., Lohr, N.E., Westen, D., & Hill, E.M. (1990), Childhood sexual and physical abuse in adult patients with borderline personality disorder. *Amer. J. Psychiat.*, 147:1008–1013.

Ogden, T.H. (1982), *Projective Identification and Psychotherapeutic Technique*. New York: Aronson.

Rinsley, D.B. (1980), *Treatment of the Severely Disturbed Adolescent*. New York: Aronson.

Schafer, R. (1954). *Psychoanalytic Interpretation in Rorschach Testing: Theory and Application*. New York: Grune & Stratton.

Searles, H. (1986), *My Work with Borderline Patients*. Northvale, NJ: Aronson.

Shapiro, E.R., Zinner, J., Shapiro, R.L., & Berkowitz, D.A. (1975), The influence of family experience on borderline personality development. *Internat. Rev. Psycho-Anal.*, 2:399–411.

Slipp, S. (1984), *Object Relations: A Dynamic Bridge Between Individual and Family Treatment*. New York: Aronson.

_____ (1988), *The Technique and Practice of Object Relations Family Therapy*. Northvale, NJ: Aronson.

Stanton, A.H. & Schwartz, M.S. (1954), *The Mental Hospital: A Study of Institutional Participation in Psychiatric Illness and Treatment*. New York: Basic Books.

Westen, D., Ludolph, P., Misle, B., Ruffins, S. & Block, J. (1990), Physical and sexual abuse in adolescent girls with borderline personality disorder. *Amer. J. Orthopsychiat.*, 60:55–66.

Zanarini, M.C., Gunderson, J.G., Marino, M.F., Schwartz, E.O. & Frankenburg, F.R. (1989), Childhood experiences of borderline patients. *Comprehen. Psychiat.*, 30:18–25.

Zinner, J. & Shapiro, R. (1972), Projective identification as a mode of perception and

behavior in families of adolescents. *Internat. J. Psycho-Anal.*, 53:523–530.
—— —— (1974), The family as a single psychic entity: Implications for acting out in adolescence. *Internat. Rev. Psycho-Anal.*, 1:179–186.
Zweig-Frank, H. & Paris, J. (1991), Parents' emotional neglect and overprotection according to the recollection of patients with borderline personality disorder. *Amer. J. Psychiat.*, 148:648–651.

INDEX